CHARLESWORTH'S
Chiropodial Orthopædics

SECOND EDITION

REVISED AND EDITED BY
LAWRENCE C. GIBBARD
M.Ch.S., S.R.Ch.

Appliance Lecturer and Tutor
Salford School of Chiropody
Salford Technical College, Lancashire

BAILLIÈRE, TINDALL & CASSELL
LONDON

First Edition 1951
(*Published by E. & S. Livingstone*)

Second Edition 1968

© 1968 *Baillière, Tindall & Cassell Ltd*
7 & 8 *Henrietta Street, London, W C* 2

SBN 7020 0233-X

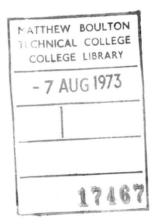

Published in the United States by
The Williams & Wilkins Co., Baltimore

Printed in Great Britain by
Alden & Mowbray Ltd
at the Alden Press, Oxford

Contents

Foreword

Dr Charlesworth's all too early death prevented him from producing a second and revised edition of his *Chiropodial Orthopædics*, a monograph which in 1951 represented a notable landmark in the development of the modern practice of chiropody. Mr Lawrence Gibbard has assumed the task of incorporating the material Dr Charlesworth had prepared for the second edition, and has also expanded the monograph by including a description of new techniques and the use of new materials. *Chiropodial Orthopædics* will thus continue to be one of the classic textbooks for all schools of chiropody.

March 1968   HARRY PLATT

Preface

THE second edition of this book presents the many advances made by Dr Charlesworth in chiropodial orthopædic techniques since it was first published, together with those techniques from the first edition which have stood the test of time. The term chiropodial orthopædics has also stood the test of time and, for reasons given elsewhere in this volume, is retained both as the title of this book and the term by which this work is known.

The various types of appliances have still, as far as is possible, been grouped according to processing techniques, and the simple devices, such as toe props, traction slings and cork wedges are retained owing to their suitability for use in School Health Service clinics. Of the more advanced techniques those which experience has shown to be of value in the treatment of congenital deformities and certain post-operative cases are retained.

Several new techniques are introduced. The most important of these is probably the moulded inlay which, with its latex plastic compound, is so simple to make up and so satisfactory in wear that it challenges the laminated surgical insole as the appliance of choice for the stabilisation of hypermobile feet. Also new to this edition are sections concerning the principles of impression taking, the use of silicone rubbers, pre-vulcanised latex, contact appliances, splint boots, surgical inlays, the elasticated moccasin, notes on leathers used in appliance making, a list of suppliers of specialised materials and the Charlesworth shoe. This latter is included to show what can be done by co-operation with the surgical shoe-maker in the production of custom-made footwear by a new method.

A new section has been included on the significance of wear marks on footwear in the chapter on shoe therapy. Although not a therapeutic matter its inclusion is felt to be justified in this chapter by the fact that an examination of worn boots and shoes gives an accurate picture of what is happening to the foot and footwear together in use. To understand this picture it is necessary to know what particular wear marks are significant in a variety of foot conditions. It is this knowledge which this section endeavours to provide. Not only can a diagnosis be made or confirmed by this means but a check can be made on the effectiveness or otherwise of a foot appliance being worn. A reduction in the severity of abnormal wear marks or their restoration to those of a more normal character following the use of a foot appliance, are an indication that the appliance is functioning properly and that the gait and stance are also becoming more normal. The material on which this section is based was originally published in the *British Chiropody Journal* and subsequently appeared in altered form in Dr Charlesworth's *Chiropody, Theory and Practice*. I am grateful to Dr Miller of the Actinic Press for permission to use the blocks of the line drawings (Figs 79–87) which Dr Charlesworth drew for use with my original article and which he used himself in his book and also for permission to use the blocks for Figs 21, 25, 26 and 28.

With care in fitting, corrective insoles and most rest appliances can be satisfactorily accommodated in normal footwear of a reasonable type, but it will be appreciated that the extra bulk involved in some cushion insoles frequently necessitates the provision of special shoes to accommodate them. As these, however, are usually made for chronic cases exhibiting painful pressure symptoms and gross deformities of the toes, the need for special shoes for these appliances cannot be regarded as unreasonable. In this respect the passing of the patient, together with the appliance, to the surgical shoe-maker for him to measure the foot on the appliance and make footwear to encompass both is the ideal arrangement.

Even although the weight of evidence has confirmed that chiropodial orthopædics is a valuable therapeutic field in its own right, the reader must be warned that its application should still be as part of a properly co-ordinated system of progressive treatment. It has been found that many of the most effective appliances are based on careful observations and experiments in padding and strapping during what one may term orthodox chiropodial treatment. In these cases appliances were introduced at a stage in the treatment when their application was likely to be most effective.

The inclusion of appliance training into the syllabus of chiropody training schools to meet the examination requirements of the Society of Chiropodists is an indication of the extent to which this work has become an integral part of chiropodial training and practice. Students will find this book invaluable in their preparation for the Society's final examination which is, at present, the only way whereby new entrants into chiropody can attain to State Registration.

Experienced chiropodists who are prepared to learn and study the techniques described in the text will find it possible to make corrective and cushioning appliances for their patients based on the same principles as the paddings and strappings they normally use. In addition orthopædic surgeons, physiotherapists, orthopædic appliance makers and surgical shoe-makers will all find valuable information and ideas which they can employ in restoring the mobility and comfort of their patients.

I am indebted to many people for assistance rendered in the production of this book. First of all to Mrs Charlesworth, M.Ch.S., S.R.Ch., at whose request I took over the preparation of this edition and who allowed me full use of the notes and revisions already made with a second edition in mind by the late Dr Charlesworth; to Mr W. Sayle-Creer, M.Ch.(Orth.), F.R.C.S., for access to case records and the use of clinical photographs of patients from his orthopædic unit at Hope Hospital, Salford, and to the British Boot, Shoe and Allied Trades Research Association for loan of the photographs used for Figs 74–77, and to Mr T. P. Bradley, F.Ch.S., Head of the School of Chiropody, Salford Technical College for the loan of photographs used for Figs 153 and 154. I am also indebted and grateful to Mr R. Smedley, M.Ch.S., S.R.Ch., for his assistance in proof reading and the preparation of the index and to many others who helped with suggestions and typing, for without their assistance this edition might never have been completed.

Manchester, February 1968   LAWRENCE C. GIBBARD

I

Introduction

IT is now accepted that chiropodists feel the necessity for a broader and more constructive approach to treatment than has been acceptable in the past.

The skilful removal of excrescences and the application of protective dressings have undoubtedly resulted in relief of pain and in temporary comfort for the patient. Such treatment, however, is of a palliative nature. The use of adhesive felt padding for corrective purposes is limited in its scope and fails in some cases to achieve its full object. Corrective padding must be applied regularly over a long period if an appreciable degree of correction is to be hoped for. It will, however, be the experience of most chiropodists, that before the desired result has been achieved, the repeated application of adhesive pads and dressings has had a very deleterious action on the skin, resulting in a plaster dermatitis or maceration.

From the point of view of hygiene, felt pads and strapping in prolonged contact with the foot are not desirable. The dressings become saturated with perspiration and encrusted with dirt from the shoes. Even with the most careful patient, padding frequently tends to become displaced to a degree that considerably reduces its effectiveness.

It is, of course, recognised that skilled reduction of callosities and enucleation of corns, accompanied by ingenious padding of painful areas, is a most necessary initial treatment in most cases, but once the preliminary treatment has achieved its object of relieving pain, the chiropodist should be in the position to embark upon a progressive line of treatment envisaging a definite end-result.

Many cases are of a chronic character and the possibility of a cure is out of the question or at least very remote, but it is in such cases that ingeniously devised appliances have produced remarkable and even spectacular results. In many cases of serious deformity of the foot, both congenital and acquired, the fitting of appliances made on the principles outlined in this volume has resulted in greatly improved stability, with consequent benefit to posture and gait and the progressive elimination of painful pressure symptoms.

The term chiropodial orthopædics is thought to be appropriate since it is already widely agreed that this work is essentially orthopædic in nature and because it is specialised to the foot and has been developed by chiropodists in whose field it lies. As such it is highly skilled and specialised work based upon a sound academic training in chiropody and a thorough knowledge of anatomy, regional surgery and foot function. Use is made of mechanical appliances designed for each patient, evolved as a result of most careful assessment of each individual problem. It covers a very extensive field and the orthopædically minded chiropodist can not only treat the minor lesions and defects of children's feet effectively by simple splint and traction devices, but achieve astonishing results in gross lesions, abnormalities and deformities in all age groups. This is achieved by the use of stabilising splinting and prosthetic devices designed for each particular patient and problem. In this field the practitioner is able to replace palliative treatment (which, although it may alleviate, does not cure), with treatment which aims at a permanent improvement in the patient's condition.

In many cases assistance can be afforded to the orthopædic surgeon to bring his work to a more successful conclusion not only by designing appliances as a post-operative procedure, but also by prior consultation with him as to the aims to be achieved so that both operation and appliance technique can be better reconciled. In other instances very successful results can be achieved where the patient has refused surgery. It is also frequently possible to obtain excellent results by the combined use of prosthetic and stabilising appliances for gross deformities and absences of a congenital nature.

The practitioner may be tempted to say that he has frequently endeavoured to treat his patients by the fitting of various replaceable devices, bunion shields, metatarsal socks and supports. He may point out how frequently the results have proved most disappointing. The answer to these observations is that such appliances are usually mass-produced to standard patterns.

The author does not deny that many useful devices have been produced by the appliance manufacturers. A number of simple shields, props, traction slings and metatarsal appliances have been introduced in recent years which have proved adequate to the needs of many patients. Various types of arch supports have been successfully fitted, but in this field the usefulness of mass-produced appliances has proved to be limited. Many have required extensive remoulding or other modification by an experienced practitioner.

In general, however, if appliances for the treatment of the human foot are to be applied with the best prospects of success, be they protective shields, rest appliances or corrective insoles, they must be individual to the patient, made on casts of the patient's feet. Only in this way will they fit truly the contours of the feet for which they are made.

Appliances of this kind are devised as the result of a careful assessment of the case. Their success is dependent upon the skill and sound judgement of the chiropodist in assessing the case, deciding upon the end-result which he hopes to achieve, and his ingenuity in devising an appliance appropriate to this end. It is this ability to assess the case and prescribe the appropriate appliance that is the vital factor, distinguishing the professional chiropodist from the mechanic.

Chiropodial orthopædics covers a wide field. It includes not only the devising, processing and fitting of all manner of appliances for defects and deformities of the feet, but it also requires the practitioner to possess a sound knowledge of shoe therapy. In many cases the basis of successful treatment is laid by the prescription of appropriate footwear. In others it may be necessary to prescribe surgical alterations to shoes as part of a co-ordinated system of progressive treatment.

It is encouraging to note that on the occasions when the author has been privileged to lecture and demonstrate on the subject of chiropodial orthopædics to orthopædic surgeons and other members of the medical profession, they have been unanimous in expressing the view that this work will supply a long-felt want.

The view has been expressed that such appliances supply the answer to the treatment of many minor deformities of the feet, in which surgery is contra-indicated, or not acceptable to the patient. Also, in certain cases these appliances enable the patient to benefit more effectively from surgical treatment.

Surgeons are particularly impressed by the great accuracy in the fit of appliances processed by these techniques, and endorse the importance of individuality in surgical appliances. It cannot be over-emphasised that appliances of the nature outlined in this volume can also greatly assist physiotherapists in the treatment of their patients. It is hoped that in this work a common ground for co-operation between the chiropodial orthopædist and the physiotherapist will have been established. In combination, these two important supplementary medical professions can be extended, and can improve their service to humanity as part of the Orthopædic Services under the guidance and direction of the orthopædic surgeons.

B

2

Impression Taking and Casting

I T will be readily appreciated that for most appliances designed to correct defects of the feet or to protect painful prominences, plaster casts provide the only reliable basis upon which to build. An accurate replica of a foot, or part of a foot, for which an appliance is to be designed, will enable the chiropodist to produce a device that will embrace the contours accurately. In this way the individual characteristics of the human foot are taken into account, with a degree of perfection not possible by any other means. As a basis for corrective and palliative appliances, our requirements in the matter of casts will be very considerable. We may require a cast of the whole foot, possibly including the ankle for certain corrective devices, whereas for surgical insoles plantar casts are all that is required in most cases. Many appliances, however, will require the cast of only a small area of the foot, e.g. protective shields for bunion, or for calcaneal exostosis, and the smallest casts are those for defects of the lesser toe. In taking casts of the toes for protective shields it is important that this should be done with the toe held at the same angle to the foot as it would assume in the patient's normal shoe, the angle being determined by the height of the heel and consequent pitch of the shoe. The taking of plantar casts first involves a negative impression which is then filled with plaster of paris to produce the positive cast. When possible, it is advisable to use superfine dental plaster for this work.

PLASTER OF PARIS

Plaster of paris has been in use for one purpose or another for over 2000 years. It derives its name from the fact that it is made from a product of gypsum mined in the quarries near Paris.

It is one of the most important materials used in orthopædic surgery and is essential to the dental surgeon. Of recent years, however, plaster of paris has come to assume an important rôle in the practice of some chiropodists, and there is no doubt that in future years it will be as important in this profession as it is in surgery and dentistry.

The manufacture of plaster of paris has improved very greatly during the past few years. At one time it was very impure, which caused much trouble in mixing, in obtaining the correct consistency and in rate of hardening.

The materials as mined and used in dental plasters are 95 per cent. gypsum, the impurities being natural anhydrites, carbonates, rubidium oxide and some silica. These impurities have little or no effect on the physical properties of the materials and act only as adulterants.

The setting times of plaster are controlled by several factors: quality of manufacture, spatulation, plaster–water ratio and by the addition of substances to accelerate the setting.

Manufacture

Should soluble anhydrite be present as an impurity in a considerable quantity, a decrease in the setting time of the plaster will result.

Spatulation

It may be accepted that, within certain limits, the more thorough the spatulation of the plaster–water mixture, the quicker it will set.

Plaster–Water Ratio

The greater the proportion of plaster to water, the shorter will be the setting time.

Assimilation

The rate of setting may be speeded up by the addition of common salt, about a teaspoonful to a foot cast will be adequate to speed up the poorer plaster, but the superfine dental plaster as a rule sets with adequate speed to meet the requirements of the chiropodist without the addition of this ingredient.

Plaster Mixing

If good casts are to be obtained, it is necessary to acquire the ability to mix the plaster of paris to the correct consistency. Although instructions, either written or verbal, are necessary to convey essential basic information, only diligent practice will induce the required skill.

Plaster of paris may be mixed in any suitable receptacle, but a rubber plaster bowl is particularly useful as any surplus of solid plaster can be easily removed after casting, and disposed of in the waste-bin.

It is not possible to be exact in the matter of quantities when advising a plaster mixing, owing to the considerable variation in qualities of plaster. It should also be noted that atmospheric variation can affect the mixing and setting. It will, however, be useful to note that approximately one quart of water will absorb about four pounds of superfine dental plaster, producing a full-bodied cream that will pour freely yet set quickly into a pot-hard cast. A little experimenting will enable the practitioner to ascertain the approximate quantities of plaster and water required for each type of cast. If these quantities and other relevant points are noted, a table can be prepared to which reference can be made and much time and material saved in consequence; the ratio is approximately two fluid ounces of water to three ounces of plaster by weight.

When plaster is being mixed, one method is to place the water in the bowl first and to sift the plaster gradually into it, the mixture being stirred thoroughly all the time to avoid clotting and lumpiness. If stirring is continuous and mixing thorough, the result should be a smooth cream. Setting can be speeded up by the addition of a little salt—about one tablespoonful to a quart of mixture.

Another method of mixing the plaster is to place the measured amount of water in the bowl, and then to sift in the plaster and allow it to settle to the bottom. Plaster is added until the water has taken as much as it can absorb. The mixture should be allowed to stand for a few minutes, after which a layer of surplus water will be noted. This water should be carefully poured off and the remaining plaster-water content of the bowl briskly spatulated until it assumes the consistency of cream. As plaster deteriorates quickly in the presence of damp, it should be stored in a metal container with a tight-fitting lid and kept in a dry place.

SEPARATING MEDIA

When taking a plaster of paris negative using the bandage technique or the plaster technique, a separating medium is used first on the skin to prevent the plaster adhering to it, and then on the surface of the negative cast to ensure the easy separation of the positive.

There are a number of separating media used for this purpose. Petroleum jelly is frequently used, in which case care should be taken to ensure that only a thin even film is applied.

In the case of the negative mould the lubricated surface should be passed through the flame of a spirit lamp or Bunsen burner to melt the jelly and ensure its even spread. When small and inaccessible areas are to be lubricated a light machine oil can be used. This should be swilled round in the cavities and then drained off.

Another separating medium is a thin soap solution. This is a very satisfactory separating medium and is applied by dipping or with a soft brush. This leaves a fine film on the surface of the negative mould that is so slight as to have a negligible effect upon the accuracy of the cast.

Sodium silicate (water-glass) is also a good separating medium which can be painted over the surface of the mould leaving a fine, smooth surface.

Another separating medium is now available which has, to a very large extent, overcome the shortcomings of petroleum jelly, light oil and soap solution. This is a 1 per cent. solution of sodium alginate. It is used in exactly the same manner as the other separating media. It is a thin syrupy solution which is poured into and out of cavities in a negative cast or brushed onto flat surfaces. It is also brushed onto the skin before the application of plaster of paris to it. On the setting of the plaster it is found that this solution has become a thin papery film of sodium alginate between the surfaces which separate readily. It is too fine to obliterate surface detail so that skin wrinkles, hair and striation patterns can be readily distinguished on the final positive. The solution can be purchased ready made up from dental suppliers, but should the sodium alginate powder be purchased it is best dissolved by sprinkling a little at a time into a bowl of water, stirring vigorously meanwhile, until dissolved.

It is not necessary to use a separating substance on the skin with impressions with dental compound, dental wax or alginate casting compound, but the use of 1 per cent. sodium alginate solution is recommended whenever plaster of paris is to be brought into contact with the skin.

NEGATIVE IMPRESSIONS

The negative impression supplies the contours of the object to be reproduced in reverse and is the mould into which the plaster is poured to produce the positive cast. A considerable variety of materials can be used for the taking of negative impressions, particularly impressions of small objects such as toes, joints, etc. For the large casts such as a full foot, a plaster negative is sometimes used, but the introduction of plaster of paris bandages as a successful means of negative casting has resulted in a considerable reduction in the popularity of negative casting with loose plaster of paris.

Casting with Plaster Bandages

Casting a foot by plaster of paris bandages is usually referred to as slipper casting. The layers of bandage are applied over the foot to form a thin, firm shell. When set, this is cut down the dorsum with plaster scissors and removed like a boot or slipper, hence the name which has become associated with this method. The slipper casting method is also used for the more shallow foot casts, and it would be appropriate at this stage to mention that a particular make of plaster of paris bandage, Gypsona, is greatly superior to the old-fashioned plaster of paris bandages made by patting plaster of paris into loose gauze bandages. The binding medium in the bandage fixes the plaster firmly in it before washing, does not interfere with the softening when it is immersed in water, and yet assists in retaining it in the texture of the bandage.

The Gypsona bandage can also be used to make negative casts of small areas by applying a number of pieces of appropriate size and shape to build up a mould of adequate strength. As in slipper casting, this plaster and gauze shell is used as a mould from which the positive cast is made. A little red or yellow ochre mixed with the plaster forming the positive cast will assist in distinguishing the cast when the bandage forming the negative is removed.

Putty Casting

Plantar casts can be made by the putty casting technique. This method, originally introduced by the author, consists of using a slab of plumber's putty into which the sole of the foot is pressed to provide the plantar impression. This impression also acts as the mould into which the plaster is poured in the making of the positive cast.

Dental Composition and Dental Wax

Other useful media for taking impressions of small objects are dental composition and dental wax. The lesser toes, individually or collectively, bunions or exostoses, are the most suitable subjects for casting with these materials. When cold, the composition is hard and brittle, but softens to the consistency of putty when immersed in hot water. It is supplied in cartons containing a number of small slabs of about $\frac{1}{4}$ inch thickness. When softened by immersion in the hot water the material is readily moulded to the contour to be cast, and sets very rapidly into a hard and brittle shell. Dental wax, which is produced in thin sheets approximately $3\frac{1}{2}$ inches by $7\frac{1}{2}$ inches and packed in cartons of about fifty, is a very suitable, if delicate, medium for toe casting. Great care is required in its use as it is fragile and easily distorted.

ALGINATE CASTING COMPOUND

An excellent material for the taking of impressions of small objects is alginate casting compound.

There are many of these compounds now on the market which were originally intended for dental casting. They are made from extractions of certain kinds of seaweed and when mixed with water jell to form a flexible mould of great accuracy. So exact is the impression that all skin creases and hairs are reproduced in the positive cast.

Another important feature of this material is its flexibility, which is such that the removal of the mould from bulbous-ended toes, toes with deflected terminal phalanges and even the gross deformity of a severe hammer toe, is possible in one piece and is a distinct advance on other methods of toe casting. It is too expensive for use in full foot casts except where they are required for exhibition purposes or for models in teaching.

It should however be noted that alginate compound requires great care in its preparation, but as comprehensive instructions are provided with each container this should not present any serious difficulty.

Impressions should be filled with plaster of paris cream fairly soon after being taken. If this cannot be arranged they should be kept moist as drying out will cause distortion.

PRINCIPLES OF PLANTAR IMPRESSION TAKING

Since, to carry out its proper function, the foot is called upon to act in turn both as a static support to the body and as an active performer in moving the body about, there is a certain amount of difficulty in deciding as to which function should be accorded most importance when taking an impression of the foot upon which to build an appliance.

The historical background is that at first impressions were taken under non-weightbearing conditions, but so many allowances had to be made for the expansion of the foot and movement of soft tissue under pressure that impressions began to be made under full weightbearing. These impressions were static and made no concessions to movement, so methods were sought which would allow for a moving or dynamic impression being made. One of the early dynamic methods was evolved in Germany whereby a compound which was capable of being softened by warming was made up as a blank insole. This was warmed and inserted in the shoe. The patient then wore the shoe, walking about until the insole cooled. This insole then took an active or dynamic plantar impression which became the actual appliance. About the same time as the dynamic approach was being worked out the author of this book evolved his semi-weightbearing method employing a tray full of putty so that impressions could be taken incorporating correction applied to the foot itself during the actual taking of the impression.

The Americans took over from here and developed several methods of making dynamic inlays inside the shoe by means of thick paste impression compounds which, again, when hardened off became the basis of the shoe inlay. Whichever method is used we cannot get away from the fact that the sole of each foot has in turn to support the whole body weight, and that whatever impression method is used we can only deflect weightbearing pressures from one part of the foot to another and unless a stick, crutch or some other walking aid is used, we cannot reduce the total load on the foot. In fact in so far as the appliance has any weight we can only increase the total load, for, as each foot is lifted, the weight of the appliance in that shoe is added to the weight to be sustained by the opposite foot. Since we cannot reduce the total load we must redistribute it according to two principles. One is that the patient shall be comfortable, i.e. with pain and discomfort being relieved. The other is that the distortions and deflections of the foot due to weightbearing shall be prevented or corrected. It is of course essential that the footwear shall be able to accommodate both the appliance to be made and the foot. This last factor often leads to such modifications of the appliance as to nullify to a large extent its effectiveness. The footwear is very often our greatest handicap.

It has been the experience of the compiler of the second edition of this book that, while there is room for all three of these methods of impression taking, the method to be selected for any individual patient requires a careful preliminary assessment of what it is expected to achieve together with what is considered will be possible in view of the patient's activities and the footwear habitually worn. The conditions under treatment must also be considered from the aspect of whether they are static or active (dynamic) in origin. Static conditions naturally require a static impression but the converse, that active conditions require a dynamic impression taken in the shoe, is not altogether correct. It is not such a simple problem as that because a foot under active conditions stretches by elongating and widening. It also distorts and deflects until it gravitates into a rigid position and is held in that position by tight internal structures or by a compressive external resistance arising from the shoe or the ground. Normally elements of both contribute to the ultimate stability of the foot. If the foot functions normally there is no complaint of pain from tight internal structures or of pain from ground or shoe compression; neither is there any weightbearing deflection of the foot. We do not usually see feet like this and therefore tend to lose sight of the normal healthy criteria of good function allied to correct shoe fitting. Our patients all have some pain or foot deflection on weightbearing. They often have both and our task is to bring relief. It is necessary therefore to decide upon the method of impression taking as part of the overall treatment of the patient.

The non-weightbearing method is really only suitable for patients with quite stiff rigid feet which do not elongate on weightbearing and it matters little whether the impression is taken with plaster of paris, either the cream or the bandage, or in a tray of impression compound such as Plasticine or putty. The plaster of paris bandage method is normally used when a deep cast is required to include the dorsum of the foot and perhaps the lower parts of the leg. These casts would be required for making moccasin appliances or surgical shoes. If plantar impressions only are required, a tray of putty or plaster of paris cream will suffice.

The semi-weightbearing impression has advantages which may not be fully appreciated. The main one is that the position of the foot can be manipulated during impression taking so that weightbearing deflections do not occur and varying degrees of correction can be applied at different points, i.e. at the levels of the ankle, sub-talar and mid-tarsal joints. It is for this reason that it is my choice where pronation defects occur in feet of any age. Here the deflection takes place at any of the above-mentioned joints and, by inverting the heel and everting the forefoot and by pressing the ball of the great toe down into the impression compound, a corrected impression of the foot is obtained, the degree of correction is under complete control and so is the extent to which it is applied to any particular joint or joints. Another advantage of this method is that an appliance made on a cast of the foot taken before it reaches full stretch will prevent the foot from stretching fully under weightbearing and so relieve pain arising from tension on internal structures.

Correction of this kind can only be applied to a foot in which there is still movement in the joints. Many feet have too much movement which the leg and foot muscles are unable to control effectively. These hypermobile feet are the ones which do best on appliances made to a plaster cast, the impression for which was made semi-weightbearing, with correction applied during the taking of the impression. In wear the foot is held stable on these appliances and tensions on both ligaments and muscles are avoided. Since the foot is held in a corrected position it cannot deflect under weightbearing so much as formerly, if at all. Consequently muscles can apply their entire effort to propulsive action and excessive fatigue arising from the need to hold the foot steady under weightbearing is avoided.

It would appear from first glance that the active or dynamic method of taking impressions within the shoes attains to the ideal. It has several important advantages. First of all it results in an impression of the plantar aspect of the foot under functioning conditions. It also provides an accurate impression of the sole of the foot and fills in the space between the foot and the shoe. As a result the appliance is bound to go in the shoe without needing modification. This ensures that its fit is not disturbed and its character is retained. Possibly its greatest advantage is that the impression compound upon curing or hardening becomes a firm resistant structure which can be finished off with the minimum of laboratory procedures.

There is, however, sometimes a little difficulty in handling this method owing to the limitation of access imposed by taking an impression in the shoe. Also paste compounds even when inserted in a well fitting insole tray and covered with polythene sheet become extruded under pressure into the shoe, entailing considerable cleaning up afterwards. Wool felt insoles soaked in thick latex or into which latex paste or butter is firmly rubbed before insertion seems less objectionable in this way, and the method whereby a thin compressible rubber sheet insole (Molo) is employed is exempt from this criticism as are thin insoles cut from expanded polystyrene sheet. The final point which merits mention is the principle on which this method works. It is essentially a displacement method in which the foot sinks into a compressible or dispersive medium, so that it accommodates itself in its distorted or deflected position within the shoe much as it would if the impression medium were not there. Plantar protuberances, for instance, will sink through until they come in contact with the sole and an elongating foot will be allowed to stretch to its limits. Semi-plastic impression material will be forced up into the non-weightbearing areas of the shoe, filling them until contact is made with the sole of the foot. Even if the impression compound is sealed in a plastic envelope, the relative positions of all parts of the foot under weightbearing will not be improved upon although in this instance the bony plantar protuberances may not sink right through the compound. Undoubtedly filling up of the shoe spaces increases the ground contact area of the sole and reduces its loading per unit area. This will naturally relieve painful plantar lesions of some pressure but this state of affairs can only occur with the foot at full stretch. Under these conditions pain experienced in the internal foot structures under tension cannot be expected to be greatly relieved, nor can a great deal of improvement be expected in muscular function. It is difficult also to correct weightbearing deflections by this method. Nevertheless this method has its devotees who use it successfully for many foot conditions. It proves also to be an admirable method particularly where patient co-operation in the footwear problem is not as full as one would wish. The dynamic method, giving as it does an exact impression of the sole of the foot and of the inside of the shoe, makes an excellent base upon which to build in order to obtain additional protection by means of grinding out hollows or building up. Corrective additions can also be made underneath the insole so that the close contact of the upper surface to the foot is not disturbed, although these are more effective when placed on top of the insole in closer proximity to the foot.

In conclusion then, static non-weightbearing impressions give best results with rigid feet which need soft cushioning appliances to relieve the pain of superficial plantar lesions. The semi-weightbearing impression is best suited to hypermobile feet where pain is mostly to be found in internal structures under tension and where deflections and deformities which need correction occur under weightbearing. The dynamic impression in the shoe is generally more suitable for patients who, having been relieved of pain in the feet by normal chiropodial measures, require a light and adaptable appliance to put into their shoes to prevent recurrence of their symptoms.

METHODS OF MAKING PLASTER CASTS

Plaster of Paris Casts for Foot or Ankle

For the purpose of making casts of this type, a good foundation is a shoe-box lid or similar type of container, as it controls the plaster used for the taking of the plantar impression. The leg and foot are prepared by applying a thin coating of petroleum jelly or sodium alginate solution, particular attention being paid to the inter-digital spaces. A suitable quantity of plaster is now mixed and poured into the receptacle. The patient being seated in a comfortable and convenient position, the foot is now placed in the plaster and held still until the plaster is set reasonably firmly (Fig. 1), after which it is carefully removed. An anklet of twine is placed round the leg just above the intended limit of the plaster. Lengths of twine are attached anteriorly and posteriorly to the anklet. The anterior length is placed down the dorsum of the foot to extend beyond the toes, whereas the posterior one passes down the back of the leg to the base of the heel with similar surplus. If these lengths of twine are gently pressed against the skin, the thin film of separating medium should retain them in position. The upper margins of the cast and surface of the impression should now be smeared with petroleum jelly and the foot replaced. A further quantity of plaster should be mixed for the upper portion of the mould. As soon as the cream shows sign of thickening it should be applied to the leg, being built up into a fairly thick, even coat. When it has begun to set, before it has become quite hard, the strings should be pulled through the plaster (Fig. 2) to divide the upper cast into medial and lateral portions which, when firmly set, should be gently lifted from the leg, and the foot withdrawn from the plantar section.

The chiropodist will now have the complete negative of the cast in three portions (Fig. 3), a plantar section and medial and lateral sections. It is a good plan to stretch the skin away from the margins of the cast before it is set quite hard, thus assisting in loosening the cast from the skin. Tufts of hair on the toes and dorsum of the foot, if present, should be shaved off with a razor before casting is begun.

When the negative cast is completed, it is prepared for the making of the positive cast. A thin coating of separating medium is applied to the inside of all three sections, and the margins which fit together to form the complete mould are also liberally smeared, after which the three sections are gently pressed together and secured by binding with a length of twine or strips of zinc-oxide plaster. When the assembled mould has been secured and if petroleum jelly has been used as a separating medium, it is well to pass the hand inside and smooth off any surplus which may have been squeezed through the joints. A hole should be bored at the toe end of the cast to allow air to escape and prevent its being trapped in the mould as the plaster is poured in. The plaster for the positive cast is now mixed to the

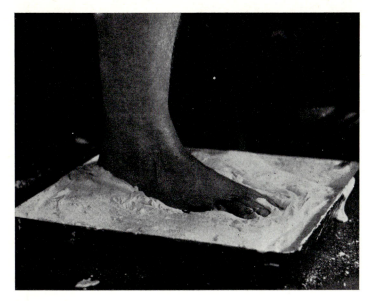

FIG. I

Plantar impression.

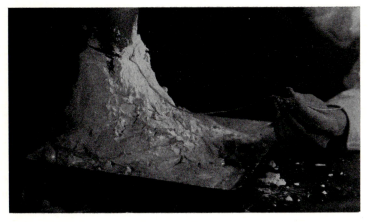

FIG. 2

Drawing the string through the plaster just prior to setting.

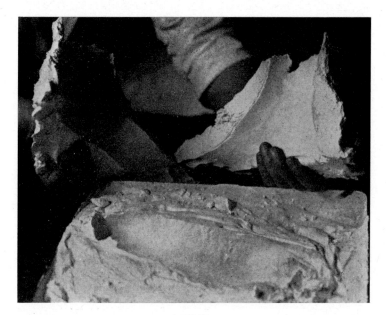

FIG. 3

The complete negative impression.

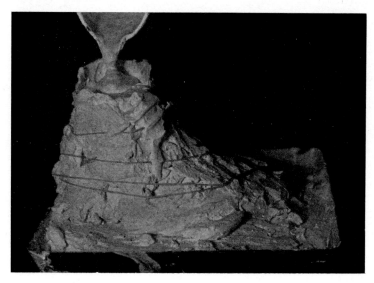

FIG. 4

Plaster of paris being poured into the negative cast.

consistency of a full-bodied cream that will pour freely. The cast should be held at a slight angle and the plaster poured in slowly until it is filled (Fig. 4). If the plaster is allowed to slop into the cast in large quantities, pockets of air may be trapped in the mould, in which case large indentations may ruin the cast. When sufficient plaster has been poured in, the mould should be shaken gently to force the plaster into every nook and corner. When the mould is filled, it should be set aside for at least an hour to allow the plaster to become quite hard. When thoroughly set, the securing band should be removed and the upper sections separated from the cast, which is now removed from the plantar section. If the operation has been carried out correctly, the chiropodist should have a perfect replica of the patient's foot and ankle (Fig. 5).

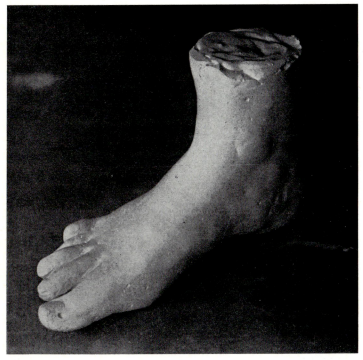

FIG. 5
The positive cast.

Shell Casting. A method of casting which produces a much lighter cast and results in the saving of a considerable quantity of plaster is the shell casting method, the technique for which is as follows:

When the mould has been prepared to receive the plaster for the positive cast, a quantity of liquid plaster is poured into it. This is now rinsed round inside the mould until it forms a thin coat over the whole inside surface. Before the plaster can set properly, the operation is repeated with a further and slightly greater quantity of plaster, providing a more substantial layer than the first. Further layers may be applied by the same technique until the plaster shell is built up inside the mould to the required thickness. In making a shell cast, great care should be taken in the mixing of the plaster, for whereas the solid cast may survive with a poor mixing, there is little prospect that the shell cast will do so. If the plaster is correctly mixed, a good firm shell will result, which will be satisfactory in every way, being both light and economical.

Small Plaster of Paris Casts

Negative impressions of small areas of the foot can also be taken with plaster of paris, this method being quite suitable for impressions of such conditions as bunion, calcaneal and cuneiform exostosis. The technique for casts of this type is quite simple, and is carried out in the following way:

A piece of strong paper of suitable size is folded into about three thicknesses; the skin over the area of the cast is lubricated, the plaster mixed to a rather stiff consistency and placed on the paper. As soon as it shows signs of setting, it is gently lifted and pressed over the part to be cast. The plaster and the foot should be held perfectly still until it is set, otherwise the impression will be cracked or distorted. When the plaster is set it should be gently removed from the foot and should result in a faithful impression of the part to which it has been applied (Fig. 6). A positive cast is now made in the way previously described.

If it is desired to take a plaster cast of any of the lesser toes, it will be found necessary to take the negative in two parts. The adjacent toes should be held away from the toe to be cast, so that the necessary working space is provided. This can be achieved by an assistant holding the toes apart with loops of cotton bandage and applying traction, but it will be far more convenient to use a simple device to accomplish this object without involving the use of an assistant. Such a device is quite easy to make and is a simple piece of apparatus.

The device consists of a board about 14 inches long, 9 inches wide and 1 inch thick. At the middle of each side are fitted posts, 12 inches in height. Holes are bored through the posts about 3 inches and 6 inches from the top. Two leather loops about $\frac{3}{4}$ inch wide are

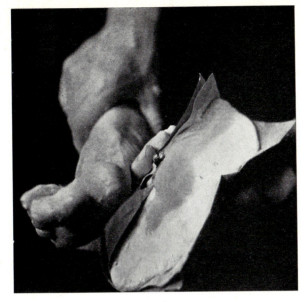

FIG. 6

Simple method of taking plaster of paris impression of a
bunion.

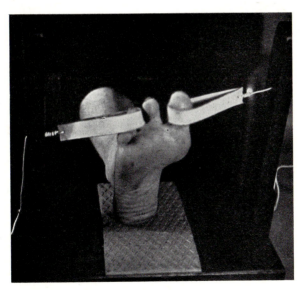

FIG. 7

Toe-separating device for impression taking.

C

made for fitting round the toes. To each loop is fitted a length of cord. The cords are passed through the holes in the post with the loops on the inside. Two notches or hooks are placed near the base of each post to which the lengths of twine can be secured. The appliance is used as follows: the foot is placed in the centre of the board, resting on the posterior aspect of the heel. The loops are passed over the toes adjacent to the one of which the cast is to be taken. The cords are then pulled through the holes until the toes are separated to the required extent. The cords are then fixed in their retaining notches or hooks (Fig. 7). In use the board should be placed on the foot rest of the chiropody chair. This will be found suitable for most forms of casting. Once again, however, it is well to remember that, when taking the cast, the toe should be held at the correct angle to the foot, corresponding to the pitch of the foot in the shoe. It should be prepared for casting by the application of a little separating medium which is applied well into the interdigital spaces and the dorsal and plantar aspects. A little tray of stiff cardboard is now made, which should be long enough to pass just beyond the end of the toe at the front and on to the plantar aspect at the back to an inch beyond the base of the toe. The tray is made by turning the sides of the cardboard up at right angles. It should be wide enough to contain the toe and a reasonable quantity of plaster at each side. About 1 inch of each side of the tray should be cut away at the rear to allow this amount of the floor of the tray to project along the plantar aspect of the foot when it is held in position for casting.

The tray should carry sufficient plaster to allow the toe and portion of the foot immediately over the projection to be pressed into it and leave at least $\frac{1}{4}$ inch clearance. When all is ready, the toe and the part of the foot involved are placed in the plaster, which should extend about half-way up the sides of the toe. The foot and tray are held perfectly still until the plaster has set hard (Fig. 8). The exposed edges of the cast are now lubricated and more plaster is applied to the top of the toe and over the dorsum to an extent similar to the plantar projection. The toe will now be completely enclosed in plaster, and this negative cast should be left in position until it is quite hard. The bottom portion is now removed, after which the dorsal half of the cast is gently lifted away from the foot. Care should be taken to see that the tongues of plaster constituting the dorsal and plantar projections are not snapped off in removing the cast from the foot (Fig. 9). The two halves of the mould are treated in the same way as the larger casts, then lubricated on the inside and on the edges and carefully fitted together.

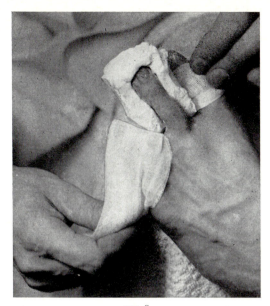

FIG. 8

Plaster of paris toe casting.

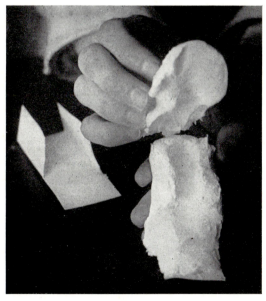

FIG. 9

Negative plaster of paris toe cast, showing cardboard
tray.

The dorsal and plantar projection portions are open at the sides, and these must be enclosed by binding with zinc-oxide strapping. In this way the mould is completed and is ready for the making of the positive cast. It may be mentioned that the small dorsal portion included in the finished cast is necessary when making the toe appliance to cover the area where the tab lies. The tab is used to assist in pulling on the appliance and securing it on the toe when a stocking is worn.

Another method of making plaster of paris negatives of the lesser toes is to fit a piece of strong linen thread round the sides of the toe and on to the dorsum, where the ends of the thread are secured by pieces of zinc-oxide plaster. The thread should pass round the toe about midway down and round the end, a little below the free edge of the nail. The tray is placed in position with some plaster already in it. When the toe has been bedded into the plaster in the tray, the remainder of the plaster is applied over the rest of the toe and dorsum. When the plaster has started to set, one end of the thread is detached from the foot and brought round the toe, cutting the cast into dorsal and plantar portions. The plaster is retained in position until quite set, when the two halves can be removed and the positive cast made in the usual way.

Possibly the simplest way of taking a lesser toe cast is to embed the toe in alginate casting compound on a casting tray. When set the compound is sufficiently flexible to allow the toe to be withdrawn, leaving the impression in one piece. This should be filled with plaster of paris cream fairly soon as the compound distorts if allowed to dry out. Piercing the tip of the impression with a sharp piece of wire before filling allows air to escape, facilitates filling and prevents air bubbles forming.

When small negative toe or hallux casts are filled with plaster of paris it is an advantage to insert a wood-screw or cup-hook into the back just before the plaster hardens. This forms a handle by which the cast can be held during trimming and by which it can be hung up to dry.

Alternatively, the base of the cast can be built up with plaster of paris to form a stand to permit latex to drain away from the main bulk of the pad during drying so that drops and runs are avoided.

Casting with Plaster Bandage

Foot and Ankle. Negative casts can be made by the use of plaster of paris bandage instead of the loose plaster. The old-fashioned method of making such bandages is to put loose plaster into open-wove-cotton bandage which has been unrolled onto a flat surface. The bandages are re-rolled and stored in a tin to exclude damp.

We have now, however, a specially prepared form of plaster bandage which is not only already prepared but incorporates a binding substance which makes the plaster firm in the bandage, and in consequence is much more convenient to handle than the bandage containing the loose powder plaster. Negative casts of a very high standard can be made by using Gypsona bandages.

The method of using these bandages is to place them in a bowl of water and allow them to soak until all bubbling ceases. The bandage is then laid round the leg in a spiral, overtopping each turn by about half the width of the bandage. When this has been carried from the ankle to the toe it is a good plan to place a plaster strip down the whole length, one from ankle to toe down the front of the foot and a posterior strip carried under the heel along the sole of the toe, overlapping the toes onto the dorsum. Another spiral of bandage can now be applied which should be adequate for the leg part of the cast. It is advisable to reinforce the sole by a further two or three plaster strips carried from about 2 inches up the back of the heel and up over the dorsum of the toes to about the same distance, and two strips should be carried from the back of the heel along the sides of the foot, overtopping the dorsum at the base of the toes. These strips should embrace the sides of the foot and overlap onto the sole.

A cast made in the way described will be just thick enough in the leg portion to be firm but not so thick as to be difficult to cut with scissors. The stirrup strips and plantar strips give the required reinforcement for the foot where the greatest weight of the liquid plaster on the positive cast will be taken. After the whole foot cast has set, it should be cut down the front with plaster scissors, when it can be eased off the foot like a boot that has had the laces loosened. Very thin strip metal can be laid down the dorsum to the toes before the plaster bandage is applied and the plaster cut over the strip with an old scalpel kept for the purpose. It is advisable when preparing for this form of casting to cut strips of bandage of the required length and number before casting is begun. The author has found that if each strip of bandage is held in the hands, extended and dipped in water before applying, the cast can be built up quite easily. The secret of getting a clean, well-defined positive cast is to see that the first layers of the negative are applied correctly. The first layer of bandage should be moulded cleanly on to the skin following the contours of the foot and then the creamy plaster should be gently massaged through the bandage so that it contacts the skin evenly.

It is this gentle creaming of the first layers through to the skin that is the secret of a good cast. If this is not done the inside of the negative will have a rough-cast appearance showing the texture of the bandage, and as a result the positive cast will reflect this indifferent finish.

Slipper Casting. If only a shallow cast is required, a slipper cast can be made, using the Gypsona bandage. It is again necessary to cut a number of lengths of bandage—4 inch or 5 inch bandage is very suitable for this purpose. The strips should be of two lengths, and about six pieces will be required for the plantar surface of the cast, which should extend from about 3 inches up the back of the heel, along the sole and over the front of the toes to the metatarsal joints; about four pieces of bandage are needed for application round the heel, along the sides of the foot to the ends of the toes. As the name of this form of cast implies, the bandage is applied to the foot in such a manner as to form a slipper. A plantar strip is first applied and then a lateral strip, the latter being brought onto the dorsum and forming a 'V' at the point where the plantar piece finishes (Fig. 10). If a square finish is desired, the lateral strip can be carried straight down the sides, the upper part of it coming onto the dorsal surface of the foot at the metatarsus and toes and the lower passing round the sides of the foot on the plantar surface. The lateral and plantar strips are applied alternately until the four lateral strips have been used, after which the two remaining plantar strips are applied to give extra strength to the bottom of the cast. When set, this cast can be eased off the foot by pulling it gently down at the heel, and when it is released it can be gently eased forward off the toes.

Forefoot Casts. Plaster bandage casts can be used for forefoot casts which are often necessary when making appliances for the metatarsal-phalangeal region. It will again be found better to use strips of appropriate width for this purpose. First a strip is taken over from the dorsum to the sole of the foot and extended as far up the foot as required for the cast. The plaster is well creamed with the fingers, particular attention being paid to the interdigital and plantar aspects of the toes. A strip is now taken round the foot and should just cover the previous strip. This is also gently worked into a smooth cream with the fingers. This is done so that the smooth creamed plaster will penetrate through the crinoline and form an even coat next to the skin, thus forming a clean and accurate mould. Two or three more longitudinal and transverse strips will complete the negative, which should be finished by gently massaging the surface plaster into a clean, smooth surface. This plaster shell will be reasonably

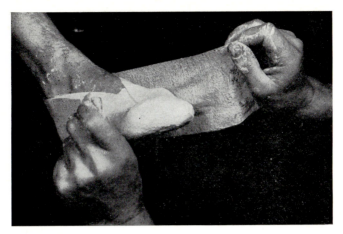

FIG. 10

Method for taking negative slipper cast with plaster of paris bandage.

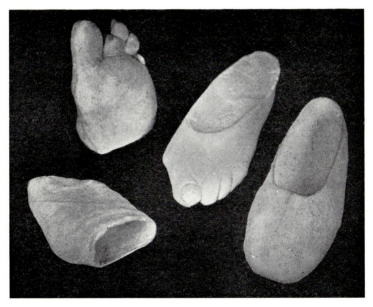

FIG. 11

Negative and positive casts (plaster of paris bandage).

strong, consisting, as it does, of firm, hard plaster interposed with layers of cotton crinoline forming a strong reinforcement. When the plaster has set hard, the skin should be stretched away from the edges to loosen the cast, which can be still further loosened by gently twisting it a few degrees clockwise, after which it can be drawn off the foot (Fig. 11).

Bunion Casts. A bunion cast can also be made by the use of plaster of paris bandage. This may be done by cutting strips each about 1½ inches wide and of sufficient length to pass from the base of the great toe round the end and to a point about 2 inches beyond the posterior aspect of the joint. The first strip is dipped in water and then placed on the outer side of the toe at its base and passed round the end of the toe to the point posterior to the joint as already referred to. This strip is gently smoothed onto the toe, and a second strip is placed along its dorsal aspect to a point level with the first strip. The second strip should generously overlap the upper margin of the first strip. When the second one has been smoothed into place, a third strip is taken over the end of the toe starting from the base of the nail over the end of the toe and along its plantar surface. This strip should be extended to the posterior margin of the first and second strips. Shorter reinforcing strips should now be laid along the toe overlying the first ones but not extending over the end of the toe. To ensure adequate strength for the joint portion of the cast, a further strip can be taken along the outer side of the toe over the joint to the base of the existing strips. This one should be wide enough to cover all the other strips over the joint but not on the toe. When this medial strip has been applied, a final strip—long enough for two lappings—is carried round the toe transversely. When set hard, this mould can be drawn off the toe quite easily after it has been gently twisted a few times to loosen it from the skin, and when removed it will be found to be quite strong. The positive cast is made in the usual way, care being taken to avoid trapping air in the toe and thus spoiling the cast. It is advisable to pierce the end of the cast to allow the air to escape as in the larger foot cast. A simpler method of taking an impression of a bunion is to be found in the section on casting with dental wax.

THE HEEL PITCH MACHINE

The purpose of this machine is to mould a slipper cast or inlay compound to incorporate the heel pitch required to correspond with the heel height of the shoe.

The machine can be used so as to produce positive foot casts which will have the heel pitch required incorporated in them so that they can be used for making shoes by a special process on the casts, as the casts can be used as models or patterns for the making of the lasts (Fig. 12).

The casts made by the use of this machine can be used for the making of surgical inlays or insoles, which will have the heel pitch and arch curve corresponding with shoes having heels of a height corresponding to the predetermined heel pitch set on the machine.

The device works in the following way:

When the plaster slipper casts have been modelled on the foot, the foot is placed on the machine with the heel on the heel platform and the forefoot on the forefoot platform, the heel platform having been elevated by the lever to the required height and fixed by the locking screw at the rear. The forefoot platform is now moved forward or backward by the handle at the front of the machine until the back edge of the platform is just behind the great toe joint.

The flexible tempered steel strip extending forward from the heel platform, and which folds down behind the back edge of the forefoot platform, will be curved to correspond with the instep. When weight is placed on the foot the slipper cast will be moulded to this curve.

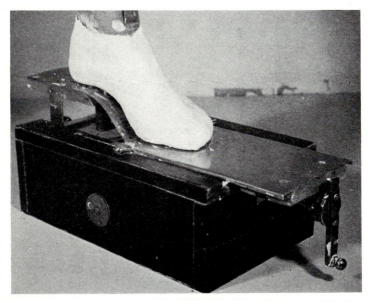

FIG. 12
Heel pitch machine in use.

The foot is retained on the machine for the necessary few minutes for the plaster to set. When the slipper cast is removed from the foot, it is a perfect negative cast from which the positive cast can be made incorporating the correct heel pitch, arch curve and forefoot spread.

The machine can also be used in the making of moulded inlays incorporating arch curve and heel pitch; it has value in research such as determining foot shortening and joint spread relative to heel height, etc. as a variety of simple measuring and calculating devices can be incorporated for this work.

PUTTY CASTING

The author has found this method, which he originated over thirty-five years ago, ideally suited for casting for corrective insoles and inlays and all forms of rest appliances.

In this technique shallow enamel trays are used, preferably one to each foot, a depth of about 2 inches being quite suitable. In each is placed a slab of plumber's putty of a size sufficient to encompass the whole plantar surface of the foot which should be about 2 inches thick whilst the quantity required is approximately three to four pounds for an adult foot which will make an impression of sufficient depth to provide for flanges.

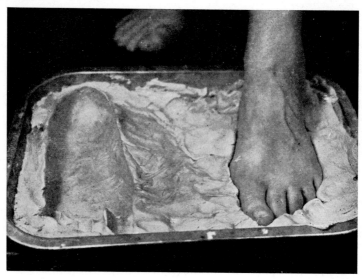

FIG. 13

Putty impression taking.

Before placing the foot in the putty the surface of the slab is sprinkled with french chalk which is rubbed lightly over the surface with the hand to produce a smooth, even, non-adherent surface.

Putty consists of whitening and boiled linseed oil. It tends to go hard fairly quickly as a proportion of the oil is absorbed by the positive cast so that the oil should be replaced at the end of a casting session. Do not use boiled linseed oil for this purpose; use the raw oil. The author has found that machine oil or liquid paraffin is more suitable for replacing the absorbed oil as it markedly reduces the tendency to harden.

This form of casting is particularly suited to the making of casts for corrective insole and inlay techniques used in the treatment of mobile pronated foot as the foot can be manipulated into correction whilst in the putty. The correction is achieved by inverting the heel and everting the forefoot, thus restoring the foot's normal arch.

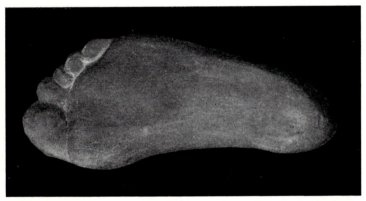

FIG. 14

The plaster cast.

This technique requires two operators, one to place the foot in position and manipulate it, and the other to press the putty compound up to the sides of the foot. The manipulation is carried out by placing the first and second fingers of the left hand in the case of the left foot on the lateral side of the heel, the ball of the thumb just below and anteriorly to the malleolus. Pressure is brought to bear to draw the heel into correction from its everted position. At the same time the head of the first metatarsal is pressed firmly down with the right hand which completes the corrective manipulation, the foot being held in this position whilst the second operator presses the putty into position. Of course, when manipulating the right foot the hands are reversed.

During the taking of the impression the patient is seated on a chair with the foot at right angles to the leg. A semi-weightbearing pressure should be exerted by the patient on the foot to achieve the necessary heel spread.

When the second operator has completed his work on the putty, the foot is withdrawn upwards, care being taken not to distort the impression.

Points to remember are: that the impression should be of sufficient depth to provide for the flanges required, and that by this technique a perfect negative of the corrected foot is achieved with a perfect reproduction of the skin texture, lesions, excrescences, painful pressure points, etc.

Plaster of paris is now mixed to a thick cream and poured into the impression. Before it has finally set, name, case number or other appropriate data can be written into the surface with any suitable pointed instrument or on a small card pressed into the surface of the plaster.

When the plaster has set, the cast can be removed by gently pressing the putty away from the sides and lifting the cast clear. The

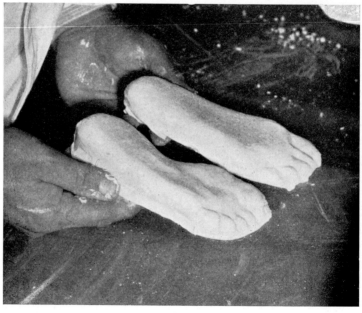

FIG. 15

Casts of corrected and non-corrected foot, nearest and farthest from the camera, respectively.

resultant cast will provide a perfect reproduction of the corrected foot. It is interesting to take a cast of the foot uncorrected and compare with the corrected one. The practitioner will be able to observe how effectively the correction has been achieved by the manipulation (Figs. 13–16 and 140).

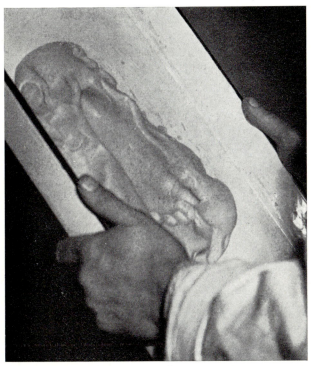

FIG. 16
Examining impressions of child's foot.

Owing to the perfection of its reproduction, putty casting is also very useful for the making of cushion surface inlays for chronic patients with rigid feet, painful excrescences and pressure areas. When taking plantar impressions of such cases, the pressure areas are frequently marked by excrescences which protrude considerably.

If these are to be adequately accommodated by cushion surface appliances, it is necessary that the impressions in which they are to rest should be adequately accommodated. They should therefore be a little over-sized to provide for the cushioning which would otherwise considerably reduce the impressions. This is particularly so if the method used is to make the appliances first and then apply the cushioning to the surface afterwards. It is therefore advisable, after dusting the surface of the putty with french chalk, to cover it with a rubber mat of the same texture as the cushioning material to be used. The mat should be slightly thicker than the material to be used for cushioning as the indentations, even in the finished appliances, need to be slightly larger than the protuberances they are to receive. The impression is taken in the normal way except that it is taken through the mat. This principle applies whether the appliance is a moulded inlay or laminated appliance.

CASTING WITH DENTAL COMPOSITION

This material is excellent for the making of small impressions, such as of a joint, one of the lesser toes or even the forefoot, but casting is more difficult on the larger areas, as the composition hardens very quickly and does not allow much time to apply it. This material is supplied in flat cakes, a number of these cakes being contained in one carton. When placed in hot water the composition becomes quite soft and can be easily worked with the fingers. A piece of the required size should be modelled with the fingers into the correct shape and then applied to the part of the foot to be cast. As already mentioned, it should be quickly placed on the area to be cast, smoothed into position and the foot held still for a short time when the material will be found to have set quite hard.

When making a bunion cast involving the great toe, the lesser toes should be held well away from the great toe to give ample working room. The compound should be pressed over the joint and round the toe and the edges brought together along the side of the toe. When set, these edges should be very carefully strained open but only sufficiently to release the toe, as the material is very brittle when set and the slightest overstrain may snap this portion off the main body of the cast. It is also as well to note that should an impression of this material be inadvertently dropped after it has set, it will shatter into pieces.

The advantage of this material for casting is that once the negative cast has been successfully taken and hardened it will not distort and will remain true to shape unless softened by heat.

A cast involving all the toes and a small part of the forefoot can be made by preparing a sheet of the composition of a length and width to enclose all the toes and the portion of the dorsum required. When heated, the material is applied to the plantar surface of the foot and pressed into the depressions on the plantar aspects of the toes. Then the composition is passed over the ends of the toes along the dorsal aspect, again being pressed into the interdigital spaces, etc. The sheet of material should be of sufficient width to allow about $\frac{1}{2}$ inch surplus at either side when it has been moulded onto the foot. This surplus material at the lateral edges should be bent at right angles to the rest of the cast so that the edges can be brought together as flanges, fitting truly to each other but not fusing. When the composition has been pressed into place and the flanges have been brought together, this cast is removed as described for the bunion cast, by straining open the edges sufficiently to allow the cast to be stripped off the toes. The edges are then brought together again and the flanges fastened together with zinc-oxide plaster. This type of negative cast does not require any lubricant or separating medium and the mould can be filled without further preparation. When the plaster has set, the compound can be softened by dipping in hot water, when it can be peeled off the positive cast. Another advantage of this material is that it can be used repeatedly. All that is required is to place it in hot water until soft and then to work it into the required shape for re-use.

CASTING WITH DENTAL WAX

This material is particularly suited to the taking of impressions of small and intricate objects. For this reason it is well suited to the taking of lesser toe impressions and impressions for bunion appliances. Forefoot impressions are successfully made by using the same technique as with the dental composition. Dental wax is made up in thin sheets and is pink in colour, and packed in cartons of fifty sheets each. When cold, it is quite hard but is readily distorted. Being in thin and delicate sheets, its application requires considerable care. Particular attention should be given to preventing distortion when removing the negative cast from the foot, and the practitioner should endeavour to harden the wax while it is on the foot by the application of cold water to minimise the risk of distortion. However, the impressions obtained by this method of negative casting are so perfect and detailed that the use of this material for small casts is well worth the extra care involved.

The author uses the following technique in the taking of small toe casts. A dish of hot water and a dish of cold water are placed conveniently beside the foot, also two or three cotton-wool swabs are laid handy. A sheet of the wax or a portion of a sheet, according to the size required, is dipped in the hot water. It is gently lifted out and laid over the area to be cast. In the case of a bunion cast, the wax is brought round the toe to the outer side, the two edges being brought together (Fig. 17). The lesser toes will, of course, have been retracted for the purpose of allowing the necessary working space. The wax is gently pressed onto the joint and onto the dorsal and plantar surface of the foot. When the wax has been carefully applied, the cold water is applied over it with a cotton-wool swab, the dish being held under the foot to catch the water as it drains off. When the wax has been hardened in this way, the edges which have been nipped together on the lateral side of the great toe are opened slightly but only sufficiently to allow the cast to be drawn off, after which they are gently brought together again (Fig. 18) and the cast is

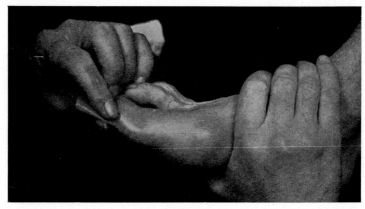

FIG. 17

Taking a wax impression for a bunion shield.

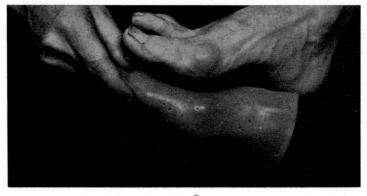

FIG. 18

The wax impression after removal from the foot.

placed in a dish of cold water which completes the hardening. Then it is removed and the surplus water shaken off. The posterior margin of the negative may be turned up at right angles so as to control the plaster when it is poured into the mould. To enable the wax to be bent without fracturing, the rear edge is immersed into the hot water to a point where the bending is to take place. This process must be done carefully to avoid distorting the rest of the cast. When the mould has been filled and the plaster set, the positive cast may be removed by dipping in hot water. The wax will soften and it can be gently peeled off. This fairly inexpensive material was at one time thrown away as it was not thought worth while spending the time necessary for preparing it for use again. If care is taken in removing the wax from the positive cast, however, it should not be difficult to reconstitute a workable sheet. The cast is placed in hot water until the wax is sufficiently soft to be peeled off without fracturing. It is again placed in the hot water and straightened out with the fingers as much as possible, after which the wax should be placed on a flat surface and rolled out with a bottle or other suitable implement. If the bottle is heated by filling it with hot water, rolling out will be further assisted. If a heated bottle is used, however, very little pressure should be applied, otherwise the sheet will be pressed out into too thin a wafer. The writer has found an ordinary cold bottle adequate if reasonable speed is used in carrying out the operation. Wax sheets reconstituted in this way can often be used several times.

Plantar impressions for sole casting can be made by using wax sheets. Unfortunately, however, the size of the sheets is too small to take other than a child's cast, and if larger casts are to be taken it will be necessary to fuse two or more sheets together. To take plantar casts by this method it is necessary to have a sheet of sponge rubber about 2 inches thick. On weightbearing, the foot sinks into the sponge rubber, and in this way the wax sheet is moulded to the shape of the sole of the foot. The wax is dipped in hot water and laid on the rubber, after which the foot is placed into position on it. Although the author has made several casts successfully by this method, he has not found it as reliable or convenient for large sole casts as impressions taken by the putty casting technique.

In taking a cast of one of the lesser toes, a satisfactory method is to cut a strip of wax of sufficient length to pass over the toe from dorsal to plantar aspect, extending it to 1 inch beyond the base of the toe. The width of the wax should be sufficient to enable the toe to be sandwiched between it and the wax nipped together along the

D

sides. The wax is softened by being immersed in hot water in the usual way; it is then laid along the dorsum of the toe and a little way onto the instep. It is then brought round the end and onto the plantar surface, after which it is pressed onto the toe, and the edges are brought together along the sides in the form of flanges. The dorsal and plantar portions of the wax should be pressed onto their respective portions of the foot. When hardened, the wax should be slightly hinged open and slipped off the toe and the edges again brought carefully together. In filling the cast the toe portion should be filled while the plaster is liquid. The wax forming the dorsal and plantar portions should be held between the pieces of cardboard, which provide a means of boxing in. The remainder of the plaster should be poured into this portion when it begins to thicken. In other words, the plaster cream should be of sufficient body as not to find its way easily through the edges of the wax and cardboard. As soon as it has sufficiently set, the cast may be laid conveniently away until it is hard enough for the removal of the wax.

Another method is to carry the wax onto the dorsal aspect of the foot, but only to the base of the toe on the plantar aspect. The toe is filled with plaster cream and as it begins to thicken it is trowelled onto the dorsal portion of the wax, being built up sufficiently thick to be reasonably strong. Before the plaster is thoroughly hard the edges may be squared up with a spatula or knife.

3

Strip Rubber Techniques

APPLIANCES made by this method are simple in construction, involving the use of latex rubber sheeting, surgical sponge and rubber solution. It is in the treatment of defects of the lesser toes in children that the author uses this form of corrective device extensively. The remarkable effectiveness of many devices of the most simple character has greatly encouraged further exploration in this particular field.

It is most difficult to retain either dressings or strappings of the orthodox materials on the feet of children for a sufficient length of time to be really effective. This particularly applies to corrective strappings. Strip rubber appliances, however, are not only easily applied, but may be removed for washing and are very durable in wear. The materials involved are no more expensive than ordinary dressings, and considering the durability and effectiveness of the appliances, not to mention the all-important matter of hygiene, strip rubber devices achieve a substantial degree of economy.

The author submits a series of examples of strip rubber appliances which have been extensively and successfully used.

Hallux Valgus Traction Sling

A large number of cases of adolescent hallux valgus come before the chiropodist. This particularly applies to the practitioner engaged in child health work with a Department of Education, although many such cases are met with in foot hospitals and private practice.

While the device described is ideally suited as a medium of correction in children, it can also be applied with beneficial results in suitable adult cases. The appliance is made in two portions, one forming a toe loop and cover for the joint, and a second portion consisting of a strip about 1 inch wide and of sufficient length to form an anchoring loop passing round the heel and attached to the base of the portion fitting over the toe and joint.

To make the toe loop, the practitioner cuts out a piece of rubber sheeting approximately $3\frac{1}{2}$ inches by 4 inches. This is shaped into an oval up to about three-quarters of its length, where it splits into two short tail pieces (see Fig. 19). When finished, this portion of the appliance should be 4 inches long, 3 inches across the broadest part of the oval portion and about 3½ inches across the tail pieces. A strip of rubber is now cut about 12 inches long and 1 inch wide. This is the strip to form the heel anchorage. To make up the appliance the following procedure is adopted. The first piece is laid on the toe with the tail pieces forward and the front margin level with the end

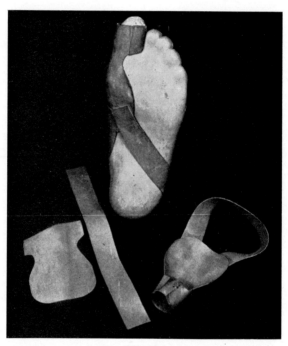

FIG. 19
Hallux valgus traction sling.

of the toe. The tail pieces are now stretched round the toe to the outside and laid one over the other. In stretching the tail pieces round the toe the degree of tension should be sufficient to grip the toe firmly. When the tail pieces have been positioned to the practitioner's satisfaction, they should be marked, the opposing surfaces treated with rubber solution and secured one upon the other. One end of the second piece which is intended for the heel anchorage is secured to the base of what now constitutes the toe loop. To secure firmly about 1 inch of overlap is necessary. When this strip has been secured in position the appliance is placed on the toe and the heel strip passed round the heel, the end being brought into position alongside the first point of attachment. Before securing the second attachment of the heel piece, the rubber strip should be stretched round the heel and held in position on the toe loop, the degree of tension being sufficient to draw the toe into a slightly varus position. The surplus rubber is cut off, again allowing 1 inch for overlap, after which the end of the strip is secured in position. Perforations may be made in the toe loop with a leather punch to assist aeration of the toe. If it is considered necessary an interdigital wedge made of adhesive felt or of sponge rubber may be adhered to the toe loop so that it helps to keep the first and second toes apart.

This appliance is suitable for continuous night and day wear, being removed at appropriate intervals for washing with a mild antiseptic solution.

Combined Traction Sling and Bunion Shield for the Teenage Child

Unlike the hallux valgus traction sling already described, the toe loop portion is anchored by a metatarsal brace and not the heel loop. A crescent pad of surgical sponge rubber is fitted on the inside of the portion covering the joint and enclosed by a piece of thin latex rubber sheeting. The air trapped in the sponge rubber by the overlying portion secured with solution forms a pneumatic padding which is very comfortable. Again the degree of traction can be determined by movement of the metatarsal brace on the foot. This device was found necessary for the treatment of the 13–15 age group where a permanent enlargement of the joint had occurred.

Traction Sling for Overlying Fifth Toe

This ingenious appliance was devised by H. A. Budin (*The Principles and Practice of Orthodigita*, Strathmore Press, New York, 1941). It consists of a strip of rubber ¾ inch to 1 inch wide and of a length ranging from 18 inches to 24 inches, the variations in width and length being accounted for by the difference in the size of foot to be fitted. For instance, a lady's foot taking a size 5 shoe, generally requires a sling about ¾ inch wide and about 18 inches long.

In making this appliance, the practitioner begins by making a 3-inch loop at one end of the rubber strip, the loop, as in the former appliance, being secured by the use of rubber solution. The loop is now placed on the toe with the short end on the underside. The rubber strip is passed across the plantar surface of the foot, behind the head of the first metatarsal, obliquely across the dorsum of the foot, beneath the outer malleolus, round the heel and attached to a point posterior to the first metatarso-phalangeal joint. The rubber should be brought round the foot with a sufficient degree of tension to exert the required traction on the fifth toe, bringing it into its corrected alignment. When the rubber strip has been brought round the foot to the final point of attachment, the surplus should be trimmed off and the ends of the strip secured in position. This, of course, is not done whilst the appliance is on the foot and the rubber under tension. It will be found necessary to cut out a shallow 'U' piece in the toe loop where it impinges upon the web between the fourth and fifth toe. This, like many other appliances by Budin, is an excellent device. It has been used extensively by the author with conspicuous success (Fig. 20). A modification of this type of appliance is to dispense with the heel anchor and substitute a metatarsal band. This merely requires the strip, after being carried round the first metatarsal, to be taken across the dorsum of the foot, passed behind the fifth metatarso-phalangeal joint, brought across the sole of the foot and attached at a point behind the first metatarso-phalangeal joint. This modified appliance may be worn in cases where the heel anchorage is not desirable. Whilst satisfactory on the whole, this modified appliance is not quite so secure as that possessing the heel anchorage, as under certain circumstances the metatarsal brace may be dislodged, with a relaxation of tension upon the toe sling.

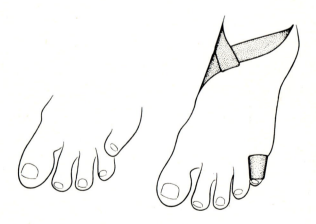

FIG. 20

Congenital overlying fifth toe (*left*); correction achieved by
use of Budin's sling (*right*).

Toe Sling and Brace for Overlying Second Toe

This is a simple but effective appliance for cases of overlying of the second toe, for which purpose it proves particularly successful. For the purpose of this appliance two strips of rubber, approximately $\frac{3}{4}$ inch and 1 inch wide respectively, are required. The narrow strip should be about 7 inches to 8 inches long, and this is used for the toe loop. This strip is looped over the toe, the two ends being overlaid on the plantar surface at the base of the toe. The wider strip should be about 9 inches to 10 inches long, and is used for the metatarsal brace. The object of this brace is to provide anchorage for the toe loop, to which it is attached by the use of solution. The brace is fitted round the foot posterior to the first and fifth metatarso-phalangeal joints (Fig. 21). The appliance is completed with a pull-on tab made from zinc-oxide strapping attached to the dorsal aspect of the loop.

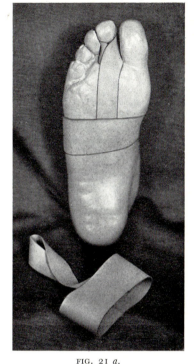

FIG. 21 *a.*

Traction sling for overlying second toe.

Traction Sling for Underlying Fifth Toe

A modification of the Budin traction sling can be made to provide traction in reverse for an underlying fifth toe.

In this appliance the toe loop is placed on the toe so that the rubber strip lies across the dorsum of the foot, passes behind the head of the first metatarsal, obliquely across the sole of the foot to the lateral side, whence it is carried round the heel beneath the malleoli and is attached at a point posterior to the first metatarso-phalangeal joint. Whilst the writer has found traction slings very effective in overlying toes, clinical observations over a considerable period suggest that splinting and propping is more satisfactory in the case of underlying toes. Peculiar features, however, do arise in all conditions when the alternative treatment proves the more successful, and it is for that reason that this device is brought to the practitioner's notice.

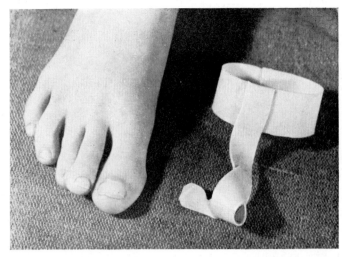

b

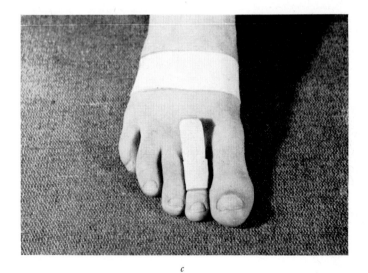

c

FIG. 21

b. Overlying second toe. Traction sling on the right. *c*. Traction sling fitted. Note the correction of second toe and improved alignment of the third.

Replaceable Bunion Shield

This is a simple device which will be found particularly useful where an inexpensive replaceable shield is required. This appliance, however, does not lend itself to being worn without hose (Fig. 22).

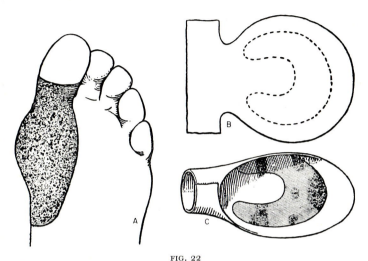

FIG. 22

Replaceable bunion shield.

To make the appliance the chiropodist first cuts a piece of latex sheeting $3\frac{1}{2}$ inches by 4 inches. This is then trimmed to an oval shape merging into two tail-pieces 1 inch wide. The approximate overall size will be: length 4 inches, maximum width of oval portion $2\frac{1}{2}$ inches, width across the neck 2 inches, total extent of tail-pieces $3\frac{1}{4}$ inches. A piece of $\frac{3}{16}$ inch sponge rubber is now cut into a crescent shield 2 inches long, $2\frac{1}{4}$ inches wide, aperture 1 inch across. The underside of the aperture is now bevelled, as is the outer margin of the shield. Rubber solution is now applied to the outer side of the shield and to the oval portion of the latex sheeting. When dry, the shield is fixed in position on the latex sheeting. The two tail-pieces are now solutioned together with about $\frac{1}{4}$ inch overlap, forming a toe loop. The measurements given are for an average size of shield. These, of course, can be modified to meet the individual case. It is advantageous to leave the securing of the toe loop until the appliance can be tried on the actual patient, ensuring a satisfactory fit.

This appliance is substantial and hygienic and its soft and resilient texture ensures comfort.

Replaceable Shield for Sub-ungual Exostosis and Sub-ungual Heloma

For this appliance a piece of latex sheeting is cut approximately 4 inches long to a shallow saddle shape. The middle third of the posterior margin should form a bulge, the total width at the greatest point being $1\frac{1}{2}$ inches. The remaining two-thirds should form two tail-pieces about 1 inch wide (see Fig. 23).

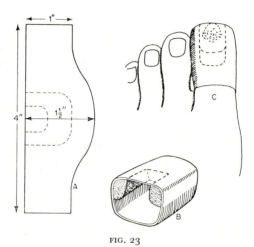

FIG. 23

Replaceable shield for sub-ungual exostosis.

A rectangular-shaped piece of sponge rubber of appropriate thickness is cut to a length of $1\frac{1}{2}$ inches and about $1\frac{1}{4}$ inches wide. The margin of one side of the pad is bevelled and a U-shaped cut-out made at one end about $\frac{5}{8}$ inch across and $\frac{1}{2}$ inch deep. The pad is latexed on the bevelled side, as is also the middle third of the latex sheet. When dry, the pad is fixed into position with the tail-pieces of the 'U' fitting flush with the straight edge of the latex sheet. The tail-pieces of the rubber sheeting are brought together and secured, with an overlap of approximately $\frac{1}{2}$ inch.

Shield for Heloma Durum of the Lesser Toes

A simple shield can be made in the following manner: a small saddle-shaped piece of latex rubber sheeting is cut, the saddle-shaped portion being $1\frac{1}{8}$ inches deep and $\frac{7}{8}$ inch across the two tail-pieces, each of a length of $\frac{5}{8}$ inch and about $\frac{1}{8}$ inch wide. A sponge crescent is cut of slightly less dimensions than the saddle-shaped portion of latex sheeting, its upper margin bevelled, and the cut-out bevelled on the underside. The shield is fitted into position and a tail-piece is secured (Fig. 24).

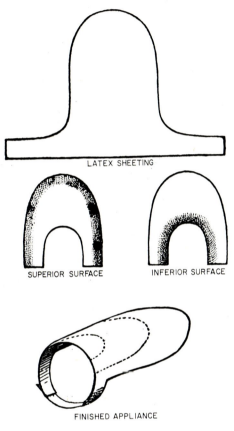

FIG. 24

Protective shield for helomata of lesser toes.

Replaceable Shield for Cuneiform Exostosis

This useful device consists of an oval shield, approximately $2\frac{1}{2}$ inches by 2 inches, with a central aperture. The shield is bevelled on the upper margin and the aperture on the under margin so that it will conform to the contours of the exostosis. The latex brace is now made $2\frac{1}{2}$ inches wide and of sufficient length to encircle the tarsus and allow for a substantial overlap. The pad is affixed centrally on the brace, and the brace secured in the usual manner.

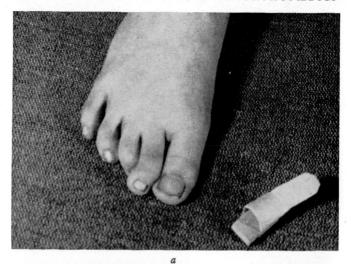

a

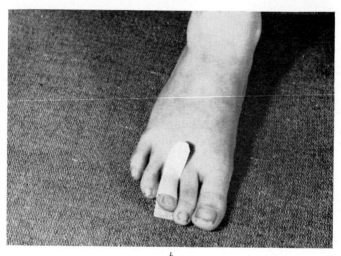

b

FIG. 25

a. Underlying and rotating third toe. *b.* Defect corrected by replaceable
toe prop.

Hammer or Contracted Toe Splint

This is a simple device and was originally made as a temporary
measure in a particular case and was found so useful and effective
that it was added permanently to our strip rubber appliances. The
splint was made by cutting out a piece from a wooden tongue
depressor found in bundles in hospitals and used when taking throat

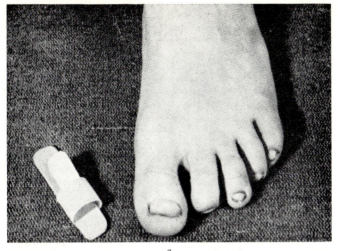

a

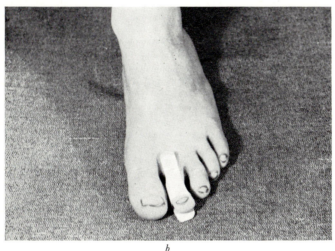

b

FIG. 26

a. Hammer second toe. Toe splint on left. *b*. Toe splint in position.

swabs and examining tonsils. This piece of thin, hard wood was found to make an excellent splint. The appliance was made by attaching a latex rubber loop and covering the splint with zinc-oxide strapping to prevent the risk of splinters becoming detached and injuring the toe. A pull-on tab of zinc-oxide strapping was also attached to this device. The appliance is simple and inexpensive and completely effective (Figs. 25 and 26).

Plantar Prop

Whilst in adults it is not usually satisfactory to extend a plantar prop to the fifth toe, it is possible to do so in the case of children when natural form shoes are worn.

A simple appliance can be made consisting of a strip of surgical sponge about $\frac{3}{16}$ inch thick and an appropriate width to fit into the crooks of the toes. As the toes shorten towards the lateral side of the

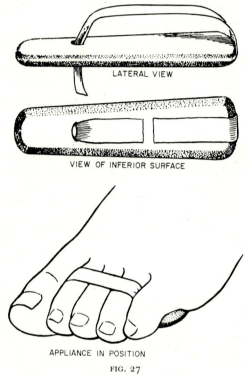

FIG. 27

A plantar prop so designed as to include the fifth toe.

foot, the pad should be correspondingly graduated in width, narrowing gradually from the second to the fifth toe. It is advisable to cut and shape the prop to the actual foot of the patient. In this way accuracy in length and width are ensured and any special peculiarities of the foot can be taken into account. The prop is secured under the toes by a rubber band, and if it is desired to involve the fifth toe an aperture may be made in the prop with a rubber punch at a point approximating to the fourth interdigital space. The band may be passed down between the fourth and fifth toes and through this

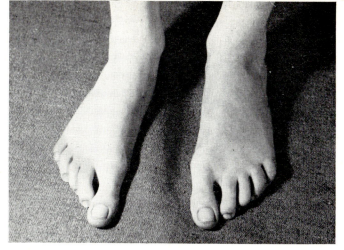

a

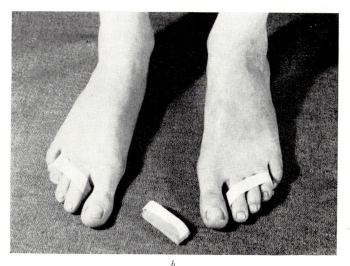

b

FIG. 28
a. Clawed toes. *b*. Replaceable plantar props in position.

aperture and attached to the outer surface of the prop. It is found that by passing the band round the fourth toe rather than round the fifth the appliance is more firmly secured and not so easily dislodged as if passed round the fifth toe. Also, the tendency for the fifth toe to be pulled under the fourth by the traction of the band is thus avoided (Figs 27 and 28).

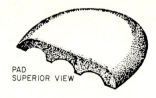

PAD
SUPERIOR VIEW

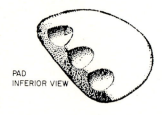

PAD
INFERIOR VIEW

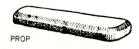

PROP

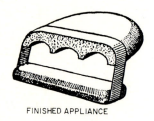

FINISHED APPLIANCE

FIG. 29

Dorsal pad and plantar prop.

Dorsal Pad and Plantar Prop

This appliance consists of a D-shaped pad of sponge rubber of appropriate size and thickness, $\frac{3}{16}$ inch to $\frac{5}{16}$ inch being usually suitable, and a plantar prop of corresponding length. The two pads are joined together by a rubber band passing round the underside of the plantar prop and along the anterior straight edge of the D-shaped pad (Fig. 29). The D-shaped pad should have a broad bevel round the posterior margin, merging into an abrupt bevel $\frac{1}{2}$ inch from the ends, where they join the anterior margin.

This appliance is more satisfactory when only involving the second, third and fourth toes. When placed in position the prop should fit on the plantar aspect of the toes, and the anterior straight edge of the D-shaped pad immediately behind the inter-phalangeal joint on the dorsal aspect.

Strip rubber appliances are simple to make and quite inexpensive, and because of this can be substitutes for ordinary padding and strapping in many instances without additional cost to the patient.

The author feels, however, that to cover all pads and props with chamois or other suitable leather will be well worth the practitioner's trouble and the slight additional expense involved.

4

Metatarsal and Toe Appliances, Using Latex, Chamois Leather and Sponge

Combined Dorsal Pad and Plantar Prop

THE materials used in this appliance are surgical sponge, cotton bandage, latex milk rubber and chamois leather (Figs 30 and 31). The appliance is of particular value because it effectively combines both the principles of protection and correction. The dorsal pad of surgical sponge is D-shaped, with a straight edge forwards. The curved edge has a long graduated bevel. The lateral margins, however, where they meet the straight edge, are abruptly curved. The width of the pad is designed to encompass the second, third and fourth toes; inclusion of the fifth toe has not been found satisfactory. Three deep flutings are snipped from the under-surface of the straight edge which allows the pad to fit snugly onto the dorsal aspects of the toes and close to the joints. The flutings leave small rubber partitions which prevent the toes from crowding and assist alignment.

The plantar prop is an oblong-shaped wedge of rubber which, like the dorsal pad, is designed to involve the three toes only. As the toes reduce in length, the prop tapers slightly towards the lateral side. In this way the difference in the length of the toes is allowed for and the prop will sit snugly in position. To make the appliance the following procedure is adopted.

A piece of fine chamois leather is cut to fit the D-shaped pad. In cutting it to shape, the leather is first folded over so that when trimmed it represents an oval and will completely enclose the dorsal pad when folded over it. The milk latex is now applied to the pad and also to the chamois leather on one side only. When the latex is dried the leather is carefully folded over the pad and pressed firmly to it. It is nipped closely round the edges, except near the ends of the straight edge which are left open. In fitting the chamois leather cover it should be pressed firmly into the flutings. The next stage is to enclose the plantar prop in similar material. The enclosing leather

E

should be of sufficient length to allow a generous margin at either end of the prop. The plantar prop is attached to the dorsal pad by inserting the ends of the chamois leather into the open ends of the dorsal pad. It is, of course, necessary to latex them before inserting them, after which the open ends of chamois leather on the dorsal pad should be pressed firmly down, completing the appliance.

Any surplus round the margin of the dorsal pad should be trimmed away. The pad is fitted by slipping the toes between the dorsal pad and plantar prop, the toes sitting in their respective flutings. The prop is adjusted beneath the toes. The dorsal pad should now be positioned with its straight edge immediately behind the dorsal aspect of the proximal interphalangeal joints.

On careful observation it will be noted that in considering the relative positions of the dorsal pad and plantar prop, the prop is set slightly forward of the dorsal pad. Combined pressure on the dorsal pad and plantar prop results in a lever action tending to straighten out the toes. The author has used this appliance extensively and it has proved consistently effective (Fig. 30). It may be noted that the device can be successfully made without involving the taking of a cast. It is, however, worth while to do so if time permits, as correct fitting of the pad to the cast during processing will ensure perfection in the completed appliance.

Metatarsal Pad and Brace

This appliance, which is familiar to all chiropodists, is frequently used to replace a similar form of padding and bracing with adhesive felt and strapping.

There are several ready-made variations of this device which function with varying degrees of efficiency. Certain facts have emerged, however, in the fitting of these pads. One is that the pad should protrude slightly forward of the brace, as this assists in countering the tendency to creep back in wear. The tendency to creep back is a common fault of this type of replaceable appliance. If the pad is extended forward with a slightly longer bevel, the foot on weightbearing would tend to anchor it. Another fact is that in severe cases of depression of the metatarsal arch, particularly in cases associated with pes cavus, the metatarsal heads tend to over-shoot the padding, which proves in consequence absolutely useless. Again, in such instances this forward extension of the pad considerably improves its efficiency.

There are three versions of this particular appliance. One incorporates the familiar pear-shaped pad, whilst the other two types

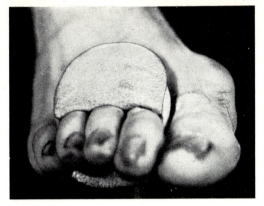

FIG. 30

Clinical photograph of dorsal pad and plantar prop.

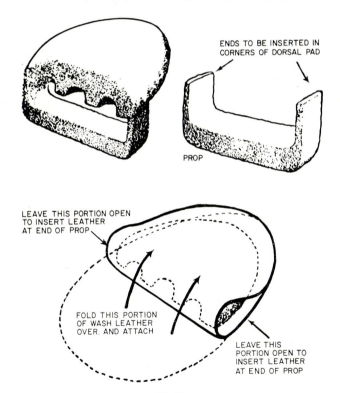

ENDS TO BE INSERTED IN
CORNERS OF DORSAL PAD

PROP

LEAVE THIS PORTION OPEN
TO INSERT LEATHER
AT END OF PROP

FOLD THIS PORTION
OF WASH LEATHER
OVER. AND ATTACH

LEAVE THIS
PORTION OPEN TO
INSERT LEATHER
AT END OF PROP

FIG. 31

Dorsal pad and plantar prop shaped and showing method of
covering.

have extensions or wings. The appliance may have a single or double extension (Fig. 32). There is yet another type devised by the author which has a forward extended bevel with toe loop. This type of appliance will be described separately, and it may again be pointed out that pads of this type may be made without the use of a plaster cast. The surgical sponge for the pad can be shaped and trimmed against the patient's foot, and the dimensions of the brace ascertained. A forefoot cast, however, will provide the chiropodist with a replica of the foot with the relevant defects upon which the appliance can be built with greater accuracy.

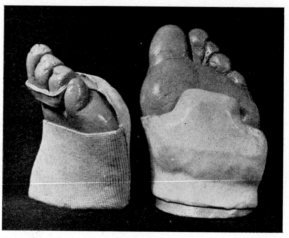

FIG. 32

Metatarsal pad and brace appliance, with and without toe loop.

In shaping the sponge rubber pad used in this device, care should be taken to see that its front margin corresponds to the curve of the metatarsal heads. Where the pads incorporate an extension it is important that these should curve snugly round the heads of the metatarsal bones they are to support. When the pad is completed, the leathers may be shaped. The material may be chamois leather, doeskin or fine basil. It is a good plan to use chamois leather or doeskin for the side applied to the skin, and the more substantial basil leather for the outside cover. Again, in fitting these leathers the sides must be left open to allow for insertion of the elastic brace.

A good method is first to fit the leather over the dorsal aspect of the pad; in other words, the side that fits next to the foot. The appliance is now held against the cast in its correct position, and the brace, the ends of which have been latexed, is stretched round the cast and the ends pressed firmly in position on the under-surface of the pad which has been previously latexed. The outer cover, the underside of which has been similarly treated, is then pressed firmly into position. By this method of processing the ends of the brace can be carried well on to the under-surface of the pad, thus securing them more firmly.

The completed appliance may now be removed from the cast and the edges of the leather finally trimmed down. Although it is not essential, a row of machine stitching round the edges of the pad makes for additional security.

The brace for this appliance may be ordinary surgical elastic or the new latex lace which is a more delicate and openly-woven material.

Metatarsal Pad with Elongated Bevel and Loop

There are certain cases where there is a marked clawing of the toes and the pain is located well forward beyond the metatarsal-phalangeal joints. At the conclusion of a course of treatment involving infra-red irradiations and breaking down of the adhesions round the metatarso-phalangeal joints, a metatarsal pad with a long bevel and forward extension, to which is fitted a loop of padded wash-leather (incorporating cotton tape to prevent stretching), will prove most beneficial. A rather large pad is made of surgical sponge with an exceptionally long bevel. Wash-leather is now shaped for the surface coming into contact with the skin. Again, basil or kid will be suitable for the outer leather. The cover is extended forward so that it comes to the base of the toes. A brace of surgical elastic is fixed to secure the pad to the foot. The wash-leather loop is now attached at one end only. It is advisable to fix the other end of the loop at the time the appliance is fitted to the patient's foot to ensure complete accuracy. The effect of the loop which passes round the three middle toes is to prevent the pad from creeping back and to draw the toes down into position. The forward extension of soft leather acts as a comforting insulation (see Fig. 32).

Forefoot Contact Appliance

Whilst the more elaborate full-length contact appliances are described elsewhere, the author feels that forefoot appliances by this technique should be placed with the older metatarsal appliances to complete the range of devices used for the treatment of metatarsal defects.

A simple contact appliance developed by Dr Herbert Prentice of New York is well worth describing as the method of construction lends itself so well to the average practitioner who wishes to confine his activities in this field to devices which, whilst being individual to the patient, can be constructed without elaborate apparatus and facilities.

The basis of this appliance is a piece of piano felt (compressed felt) about ⅛ inch thick which is cut to fit the forefoot up to the base of the toes. Two pairs of transverse slits are cut in the felt which are stretched to form loops dorsally. They are sited so as to envelop the fifth toe and the great toe respectively. This appliance, which is developed on the patient's foot, is commenced by painting the plantar surface of the foot where the felt is to fit with a rubber solution. The felt is also so treated on the surface which is to come in contact with the foot. When the solution has dried the pad is placed on the foot with the loops in position on the toes, the solution holding the felt firmly in contact with the skin.

A polythene squeeze bottle containing latex milk rubber is used in the next procedure. The latex is squeezed into the felt, gently patted into the felt until an adequate amount has been absorbed but not sufficient to overload it, in which case under pressure excessive quantities of the latex would be squeezed out.

The next process is to encompass the forefoot in a polythene sheet so as to protect the stocking which is now pulled into position on the foot. The patient is now invited to put the shoe on and walk about in the appliance for an hour or so, perhaps by going out and doing a little window-shopping, during which time the weightbearing foot in action will be acting upon the felt, moulding it to the foot and laying the foundation for a dynamic appliance.

When the patient returns, the shoe, stocking and protective cellophane sheet are removed and the felt pad will be observed moulded closely to the plantar surface of the foot up to the base of the toes. The pressure areas can now be marked with a grease pencil after which the padding is cut to provide the necessary support and protection for these areas. This may be made of felt or surgical sponge rubber.

When the padding has been cut to shape, the surface to be applied to the felt is coated with solution and left to dry. A portable hot air blower is now applied to the felt sheeting whilst still in contact with the foot to assist in the coagulation and curing of the latex milk rubber. A hair dryer may well be a suitable apparatus for this purpose.

When a reasonable amount of curing has been achieved so that there is no liquid latex remaining to squeeze out, the surface of the felt is again painted with rubber solution and when sufficiently dry the padding is pressed in position upon it. By now the moulded shield will be sufficiently cured to retain its shape and can be carefully removed from the foot. It is now placed at one side to cure after which the final trimming and shaping of the pad is carried out including the scouring and bevelling of the edges and the padding.

It will be found when the pad has been removed from the foot that the solution and any latex which may have escaped and adhered to the foot can be easily removed. The pad may be completed by covering the surface to fit next to the foot with a suitable material. My American colleague uses a soft flesh-coloured fabric. In Britain many practitioners may well favour surgical chamois leather. The appliance is completed by covering the outer side with a fine glove kid or some other suitable leather in an appropriate colour.

There is no doubt from the evidence available that Dr Prentice has consistent success with this particular device which is extremely neat and convenient for any type of footwear. The author has since produced a modification of this appliance in which a single toe loop is used passing round the three middle toes. The loop is not part of the original felt but may be made of tubular gauze into which has been drawn a strip of foam rubber. The latter should be of sufficient length to encompass the dorsal aspect of the three toes and also the interdigital aspects of the outer ones leaving two flat tags to be secured to the felt, the felt being shaped to fit up to the base of the toes.

An alternative to this is to cut a similar length of chamois leather of sufficient width to double over. A strip of cotton bandage of the same length and half the width is cut and a piece of latex foam of the appropriate length is also prepared. Rubber solution is applied to one side of the chamois leather and also to the cotton bandage. When dry, the cotton bandage is secured to the chamois leather along one side of it. The latex foam is also solutioned and when ready placed in position. The strip of chamois leather is now folded over encompassing the foam rubber, being pressed down at the two ends into flat strips. This cushioned loop is fitted round the toes and onto the felt in the same way as the tubular gauze loop previously described. It has no special advantage in efficiency over the gauze loop but its finish matches up rather neatly with the chamois leather surface of the appliance.

The author has also tried successfully a technique in which the felt is treated with a hot air dryer until the curing is well advanced, after which the appliance is removed from the foot and completed immediately. It is placed back in position on the foot and the patient leaves the surgery wearing the appliance. The final curing is completed during wear. This has been found perfectly satisfactory but it is advisable to advance the curing considerably before applying the finishing leathers.

A very simple form of forefoot contact appliance brought to my notice by Dr Martin Cole of Toronto, Canada, will probably be found the most convenient form of forefoot appliance being devoid almost entirely of any complications.

The materials used are $\frac{1}{8}$ inch and $\frac{1}{16}$ inch Molo, which is a mouldable rubber sheeting (Chapter 10). A paper pattern of the insole of the shoe should be obtained; Dr Cole uses standard paper insoles in three or four basic sizes. It has been his experience that one of them will be a sufficiently near fit with slight adjustment. The pattern used is of the forepart of the foot only from the toes to behind the metatarsals; in other words the whole of the sole part of the shoe.

The pattern is applied to the Molo sheeting and marked round with a grease pencil. The forefoot insole is now cut out and tried in the shoe so any final clipping can now be done to ensure perfect fit. This Molo insole is cut from the $\frac{1}{8}$ inch thickness. It is now placed in position in the forepart of the shoe and covered with a fine leather sock lining. The shoe is worn for a few days after which it will be found that a complete moulded pattern of the forefoot will have been compressed in the Molo. The device is now carefully removed and $\frac{1}{16}$ inch Molo is added where needed to provide protection and support, 'in accordance with standard orthopædic practice', in the words of Dr Cole.

Dr Cole has been using this technique for forefoot lesions for some very considerable time and has found it excellent, being unelaborate and involving the use of no special equipment. The more extensive use of the Molo technique includes the full-length contact appliances based upon the information supplied by Dr Leonard Hymes of New Jersey, U.S.A., who has done extensive research in Molo technique (Chapter 10).

Traction Toe Sling for Overlapping Fifth Toe (*after Budin*)

Overlapping fifth toe has received the consideration of a number of authorities from time to time, but experience has proved that a toe sling on the lines described by Dr Harry A. Budin, M.Cp. of the

First Institute of Podiatry of Long Island University, offers, so far, the best solution to this problem. The appliance devised by Budin is made from strip rubber, but a sling made of chamois leather and reinforced with latex and linen was made on the same principle. This terminated in 2 inches of silk elastic and a small hook; an eye to receive the hook was attached to the sling on its dorsal aspect. This appliance has been most comfortable to wear, and as a corrective measure has been very successful.

This appliance, whilst in no way deviating from the basic principles of that devised by Budin, and made from sheet rubber, has, in certain circumstances, been found more comfortable to wear, principally on account of the chamois leather next to the skin, also because the actual toe loop can be modified, and, if necessary, slightly padded at the base of the interdigital aspect of the loop.

It should be noted when making this appliance that the amount of traction exerted upon the toe must be carefully regulated. Frequently it is advisable to increase the traction by gradual stages. Satisfaction is rarely found in the use of an appliance of this nature for treatment of adults except as a post-operative measure, when the appliance will prove most useful. An appliance involving the principles of the Budin sling will as a general result prove highly successful for children (Figs 33 and 34).

Toe Splint with Heel Loop Attachment

This appliance is used for correcting an overlapping fifth toe, either congenital or acquired.

The splint is attached to the toe by an elastic loop, and passes along the plantar surface of the foot to a point posterior to the cuboid. An elastic loop attached to the base of the splint is passed round the heel. The method of securing the splint is very satisfactory, the appliance being easily and speedily fitted and not visible from the dorsum of the foot.

The device is made in the following manner:

A piece of spring steel is acquired of sufficient length to pass from the distal end of the toe to about 1 inch beyond its base. A flask-shaped cover of wash-leather or other suitable material is made. A strip of $\frac{1}{2}$ inch elastic sufficient in length to stretch round the toe and attached to the splint is procured, as is also a similar strip of elastic for the heel attachment. A good plan is to complete the appliance minus the heel attachment, fit the appliance on the toe, attach one end of the heel elastic only, pass it round the heel, exerting the required tension, cut off the required length and attach.

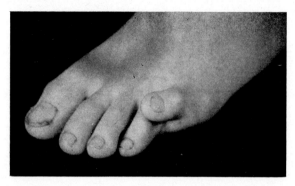

FIG. 33
Congenital overlying fifth toe.

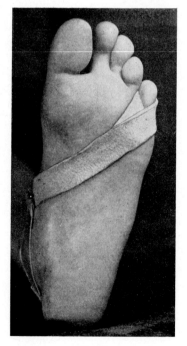

FIG. 34
A modification of the Budin sling.

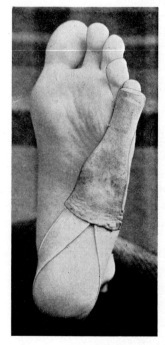

FIG. 35
Toe splint with heel loop attachment.

To make the splint a piece of flask-shaped chamois leather is prepared by applying the latex milk rubber and placing it down on a bench or table, the latex-covered surface uppermost. A piece of thin sponge rubber is now placed in position, extending from the base of the leather covering the broad portion of the flask. The metal splint is now placed in position and secured by a slip of cotton bandage previously prepared with latex. The toe loop is now fitted, the loop extending on the wash-leather side of the appliance. A flask-shaped piece of basil leather which has also been prepared with latex is attached at the toe loop and fitted firmly down the neck of the flask, but left free at the broad portion. The appliance is now fitted on the toe and one end of the heel elastic placed in position round the heel and attached as previously described. The basil leather is then pressed firmly into position.

While shaping the flask-shaped leathers it should be noted that the neck of the flask should extend the whole length of the toes and slightly beyond, the body of the flask constituting the remainder. It is advisable to run a row of stitching across the base of the leather to ensure complete security of the heel loop. Stitching may likewise be applied to the toe loop with a similar object in view. It has been noted, however, that these appliances do appear to stand considerable wear and tear even when the stitching is omitted.

When making appliances of this nature, a slipper cast of the foot is usually taken, pressing the toe in the corrected position during the setting of the plaster. The toe is also held slightly away from the fourth toe.

On completion of the positive cast the plaster may be removed from between the fourth and fifth toe by the use of a hacksaw blade. This cast provides a perfect model upon which the appliance can be built and fitted.

This appliance was devised by the author not only to bring the toe back into the normal position but also to correct the rotation (Fig. 35).

Contracted Toe Appliance

There are many cases of contracted second toe which, unlike most hammer toes, can be wholly or partially straightened under pressure. The toe when contracted brings the inter-phalangeal joint into prominence. This condition is associated with a subluxation of the metatarsal-phalangeal joint.

A simple and effective appliance for this purpose was designed by the writer many years ago. The appliance consists of a strip of spring

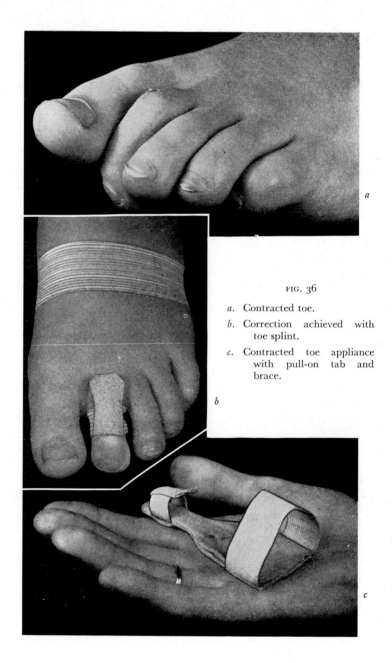

FIG. 36

a. Contracted toe.

b. Correction achieved with toe splint.

c. Contracted toe appliance with pull-on tab and brace.

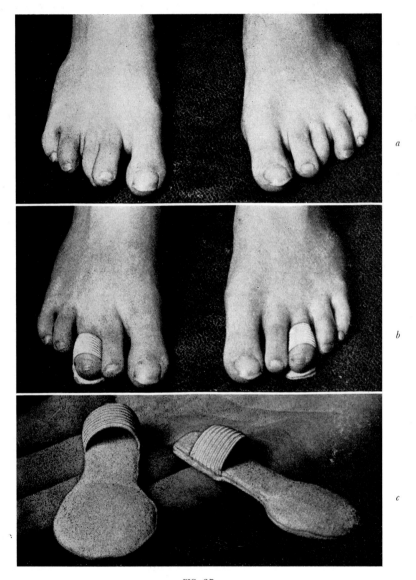

FIG. 37

a. Underlying third toe. *b.* Correction achieved by use of a banjo splint. *c.* Banjo toe splints.

steel encased in leather; the device is flask-shaped, and near the end of the long neck, which acts as a splint, is an elastic loop which passes round the toe. At the posterior or broad end of the appliance is attached a large elastic loop, which passes round the foot with its anterior margin behind the first and fifth metatarsal heads. A pocket is provided for a metatarsal pad, which may be found useful in some cases to assist correction of the subluxation of the metatarsal-phalangeal joint. This appliance is particularly effective in the early stages of the condition before any ankylosis of the inter-phalangeal joints has taken place. This appliance is, of course, constructed in the usual way. The loop may be reinforced with cotton bandage and secured with latex and milk rubber (Fig. 36).

Toe Splint without Brace (Banjo Splint)

This form of toe splint consists of a metal splint merging into a circular disc at its base, the splint stretching from just beyond the end of the toe to beneath the corresponding metatarsal head. It is the disc-like portion which is situated over the latter. The appliance is covered in wash-leather or other suitable material. A loop of surgical elastic about $\frac{3}{4}$ inch wide is fitted to the splint at a point where it will pass over the distal inter-phalangeal joint. A small tab of thin wash-leather may be fitted centrally on the loop to assist in pulling it in position. This tab should be carefully skived at the edges and should be sufficiently wide to cover the dorsal aspect of the joint so that the patient will not be conscious of any ridge. The tab is made by cutting a strip of the thin wash-leather, latexing and applying it to the elastic band by folding it over with the ends protruding to the rear. When the tab has been secured it may be finished off by rounding with scissors (see Fig. 37).

5

Silicone Rubber Techniques

An advance in chiropodial orthopædic practice has been the use of silicone rubber compounds to make permanent foot and toe appliances. By this means the appliance can be made by a process of direct moulding on to the foot so that the taking of a plaster cast is dispensed with. The silicone rubber compounds are inert and non-irritant and can be left to cure in contact with the skin at room temperatures. The compound is moulded on to the foot in the form of a paste which, when hardened, is removed, trimmed and replaced straight away on the foot for use as a replaceable permanent or semi-permanent device.

There are several such compounds on the market available as prepared rubber pastes packed in tubes or tins together with catalysing liquids and thinners packed separately. The compound is activated by the addition of the catalyst to the paste with which it is mixed thoroughly on a glass slab or in a polythene bowl by spatulation or stirring. Setting time is controlled by the amount of catalyst added. The more catalyst added the quicker the setting time. The density of the final product can be controlled by the type of compound used. Some are soft-setting, others set hard. Either can be obtained incorporating a blowing agent which turns the final product into a rubber foam.

Generally speaking foaming compounds are used for cushioning purposes and solid compounds for appliances which have to resist the pressures incurred in countering mal-thrusts. Compounds, if all of the same make, can be bonded one to the other so that it is possible to make firm appliances with soft spongy linings if need be. A silicone primer is also available for coating cloth, leather, metal or fibreglass. This permits the appliance to be mounted on a base of one of these materials.

The base is first painted with the primer and allowed to dry. The appliance is then adhered to the primed surface with a thin layer of silicone rubber which acts as an adhesive. Should any silicone rubber appliance tear or become worn in use, it can be repaired by coating the torn surface with some of the same compound as that with which it is made. On solidification the new rubber will bond with the old making an almost invisible repair. Worn areas can be built up in a similar fashion and the appliance relined if necessary. The catalyst will naturally be used in the repair mixture to ensure good adhesion and firm setting.

TOE APPLIANCES

Props

Silicone rubber can also be used to make a very satisfactory type of toe prop.

Until now the difficulty of making a toe prop to a plaster cast has been that of obtaining an impression in any but the contracted position. By the means to be described, the toes can be held straightened out by hand and an impression taken so that the prop to be made from it will keep the toes in the corrected position.

Plasticine, putty or modelling clay is modelled under the toes, corrected as to position by the operators' fingers, until the space between the toes and the ground plane of the forefoot is filled. This impression of the space is carefully detached without deforming it. The previous application of talcum powder under and between the toes ensures that it detaches easily.

This space impression is then placed in a shallow cardboard tray and plaster of paris poured over it. When hard the impression material is removed from the plaster and the impression so made is filled with silicone rubber. The grade can be selected according to the hardness desired in the final toe prop. The foaming type, either hard or soft, is desirable and plenty of tubular gauze or cotton bandage should be incorporated in the bulk of the prop.

These props lift the toes and fit so accurately under them that toe loops are not normally necessary.

Great care should be taken when making the preliminary impression with the soft material that the toes really are lifted and straightened properly. If not, these props will merely increase the curling of the toes. It is essential, of course, that there shall be room in the shoes to accommodate the toes in the corrected position.

Dorsal Toe Pads

A toe appliance to protect a painful corn can be made as follows: a single layer of tubular bandage is applied to the toe and pulled well down on to the dorsal and plantar surfaces. Two slits are required for the middle three toes but only one slit for the first or fifth toes. The tails so made are pulled back and adhered to the dorsal and plantar surfaces of the foot with zinc-oxide tabs behind the toe. Some of the silicone rubber compound is then applied to the area around and behind the corn through the bandage. A pad of foam rubber or soft felt can be incorporated in the rubber mixture to increase its bulk. While this is still tacky the open split end of the tubular gauze is twisted and doubled back over the toe to form an outer covering to the rubber. The outer surface may now have more rubber compound applied to it to make a good surface finish. Additional bulk may be added on the surface at this stage if needed. It is best to use the soft foaming rubber compound for these digital appliances and to keep the layers as thin as possible.

HALLUX VALGUS APPLIANCES

These appliances are made in a similar fashion. The tubular gauze needs to be slightly larger, say the 1 inch width, and to be at least four times the length of the toe. The thickness of the pad may be built up by making it in several layers and felt or rubber crescents can be incorporated in it. The appliance loses its tackiness in less than ten minutes. Before this time has elapsed the second layer of tubular gauze must be applied. After this time some people favour applying a layer of tubular gauze around the entire foot and putting the foot in the shoe. The final hardening-off of the pad takes another ten to fifteen minutes, and if this is done in the shoe the pad normally becomes a better fit.

METATARSAL APPLIANCES

These can be made in a similar manner to those for the toes. The large size of tubular gauze is used which can be put right round the foot if so desired. Loops are made from a smaller size of the tubular gauze to pass from the plantar pad up between the first and second toe, across the bases of the second, third and sometimes even the fourth toes and down between the toes to their attachment to the pad. The plantar pad should be built up with several thicknesses of tubular gauze to give it strength. Bulk may be increased by the addition of a pad of felt or sponge rubber previously soaked in silicone rubber before application. Here again the final hardening-off may be done in the shoe to obtain a dynamic effect.

F

Dynamic Inlays

There would appear to be considerable scope for the use of silicone rubber for the making of dynamic inlays. The rubber can be applied to a blank insole inserted in the shoe, the patient's foot can then be inserted and the patient instructed to walk on it until it has hardened. Corrective pads of felt and rubber can be incorporated in the inlay. No separating medium is required when using silicone rubber as it does not adhere to the skin, nor does it adhere to the inside of the shoe if the surface is smooth. Since some part of the inside of the majority of shoes is rough, it is advisable to powder lightly before insertion. This applies particularly to the inside of the upper which will otherwise become affected by the rubber forced out from the inlay. This method has been used successfully and the only valid objection would appear to be on the grounds of expense.

A new 'one-pack' silicone rubber is now available which does not require the admixture of a catalyst to harden it. It can be squeezed from a collapsible lead tube and applied directly to the surface on which it is to be used. As it is air-curing it should not be applied in thick layers. If it is, the centre will remain fluid and soft. The makers do not recommend this compound for direct application to the skin as it cures by an acid reaction which might cause irritation. It has been used on a tubular gauze base, taking care that the compound does not sink through the gauze on to the skin, in the production of digital pads as already described. The skin should be protected by a thick coating of tinct. Benzoin Co.

A layer of cellophane adhered to the skin with tinct. Benzoin Co. has also been employed. Some dorsal pads have been deliberately made to retain the fluid centre by applying the silicone rubber so thickly that it does not harden all through. This gives a 'hydraulic' cushioning effect which is quite satisfactory but the pad needs to be reinforced on its surface with a fairly strong material to avoid bursting. Fine nylon stockinette as used in ladies' stockings is a most suitable material.

At the time of writing, silicone rubber products show a high abrasive resistance but lack tensile strength. They are also somewhat brittle, but can be cut with a sharp wet knife. Accordingly, appliances made of them require to be filled with tubular gauze, cotton bandage, nylon stockinette, felt or sponge rubber in order to resist tearing.

Many of the digital pads, crescents, wedges and props in particular, can probably best be regarded as felt, sponge rubber or tubular cotton pads, according to the material used, which are 'set' in silicone rubber. However, this in no way detracts from their usefulness.

Silicone rubber is a useful material with many possibilities and its usefulness will be increased if it is possible to obtain improved materials with increased tear resistance.

The numbers and densities of silicone rubbers are appended here for convenience in ordering supplies. The suppliers' names and addresses will be found in the directory pages at the end of the book.

Midland Silicones Elastomers Nos. 2427 and 9161 are mixed together and catalysed with No. 2428 to make a firm resilient closed cell sponge rubber useful for dorsal digital pads as well as toe props and hallux valgus shields. American readers will like to know these numbers are equivalent to the Dow Corning Silastic No. S5370.

I.C.I. No. E.P.5708 is equivalent to Laminette reference LS and makes a soft non-foam rubber.

I.C.I. No. E.P.5688 is equivalent to Laminette reference LSF and gives a soft foam rubber.

I.C.I. Silcoset 100 is equivalent to Laminette reference LH and produces a hard non-foam rubber.

I.C.I. Silcoset 100 and blowing agent No. 1 is equivalent to Laminette reference LHF and produces a hard foam rubber.

All the above I.C.I. and Laminette numbers are catalysed with curing agent D, i.e. the ten-minute curing agent. The one-pack silicone rubber is I.C.I. Silcoset No. 151 and requires no curing agent.

6

Latex Milk Rubbers

MILK RUBBER or liquid latex is the juice of the rubber tree and is extracted by 'tapping', i.e. an incision is made in the bark of the tree trunk. This fluid contains between 30 and 40 per cent. rubber, and on exposure to the air coagulates quickly because of evaporation of the moisture. Coagulation is prevented by the introduction into the fluid of an alkaline stabilising agent, 15 per cent. ammonia solution. It is in this stabilised form that latex milk rubber is used by the chiropodist, and it is sold in this form by the shoe and leather sundriesmen and dental supply houses. If kept in a tightly sealed tin or well-stoppered bottle, latex milk will keep in good condition for about two to three months. The lid or stopper should be placed on the container immediately after use, as repeated and prolonged exposure to the air will evaporate the stabilising agent and result in coagulation and rapid deterioration of the latex. On purchasing latex milk it is advisable to see that the supply is fresh, and so ensure its keeping in good condition for a reasonable period of time.

PRE-VULCANISED RUBBER LATEX

Latex milk, whether or not it is concentrated to 60 per cent. rubber content for more economical transport, is essentially natural or raw rubber and when dry the rubber deposited is of the 'crepe' variety.

There are now available several prepared latices which are, in fact, pre-vulcanised. This means that when they dry the rubber deposited is of the vulcanised variety. Curing takes place on drying at room temperatures and no heat need be applied. These latices produce a more durable rubber deposit which is usually more resistant to friction and deformation but may have a slightly reduced tear resistance when compared with raw rubber latex depositions. On the other hand foot appliances when made from pre-vulcanised rubber do not develop the tendency to tackiness when subjected to the hot and humid conditions of the foot inside the shoe which so often spoils those made from raw latex.

The rubber deposited from pre-vulcanised latex is opaque and can be obtained coloured flesh pink. This type of rubber latex probably makes the best all-rubber digital devices but is inferior to the raw variety as an adhesive and as an intermediate dip between the lining and covering leathers of chamois-covered toe pads and hallux shields.

Should the chiropodist desire to dilute either type of latex, this can be done by adding some 15 per cent. ammonia solution. The latex may be applied by a variety of methods, namely dipping, brushing on or spraying.

Dipping

When the dipping method is used, the cast should be carefully prepared. Some practitioners prefer to coat the cast with a sealing substance such as shellac varnish, cellulose cement, or plastic emulsion paint. Another method is to immerse the cast in a weak acid solution and not remove it until all bubbling has ceased and the cast is absolutely saturated. It is claimed that this method prevents the formation of air bubbles between the latex and the cast and gives a firmer skin.

The prepared cast is immersed, apex first, in the milk rubber and gently moved about so as to ensure a thorough coating, after which it is placed to dry, apex uppermost. By placing the cast in this position any remaining surplus of latex will flow back over the whole area of the cast. Each coat is dried and the dipping repeated until a sufficient number of coats have been applied to build up to the required thickness. Usually ten to twelve coats are adequate.

Padding may be introduced in the form of felt or surgical sponge rubber, the latter is most favoured, although soft felt has proved quite successful. The padding is introduced after the application of four or five coats of the latex milk. When the padding has been carefully fitted and appropriately shaped, the remaining coats of latex are applied, enclosing the padding as part of the main structure. Padding is adhered with rubber solution, and all exposed surfaces must be sealed with rubber solution before dipping continues to prevent the latex from soaking in and making the pad hard.

Brushing On

For this method a small brush with soft but firm bristles is used—for a small cast a $\frac{1}{2}$ inch flat brush is suitable. A dish of soap solution made by dissolving powdered soap or soap-flakes in water is required. This solution is used to prevent the bristles' becoming clogged together with coagulated latex by giving them a thin film of soap. It is advisable to have another dish of clean water in which to rinse the brush out after each application of latex, the process being as follows: dip the brush in the soap solution, shake gently, dip in the latex milk, brush briskly over the cast, place the cast to dry, rinse brush thoroughly in water. To repeat the application of latex milk, again dip the brush in soap solution, carry on as before. When the final coat has been applied, thoroughly rinse out the brush in clean water.

A Simple Expendable Brush

In spite of the use of soap solutions the brush tends to become clogged so an expendable brush is really needed. A good one can be made by drawing a sufficient number of pieces of sisal cord through an 8-inch length of stout laboratory rubber tubing. The free ends, cut short and even, are then frayed out to form a brush. After use the residual latex is allowed to harden in the brush head. When it is next required for use more of the sisal cord is drawn through the tube, the hardened end is cut off and the cord frayed out again to make a fresh brush. The number of times this can be done is only limited by the length of cord threaded through the rubber tubing. An excess length of cord hanging out of the opposite end of the tubing from the brush head makes a convenient loop by which to hang the brush up to dry after use.

Spraying On

This method ensures an even coating of latex and is very satisfactory providing that great care is taken to prevent the jet of the spray from becoming clogged with coagulated latex. It is advisable to pass some 15 per cent. ammonia solution through the spray immediately after use, and to finish by using a liberal quantity of clean water. When the laboratory is organised for the processing of a considerable quantity of latex appliances, the milk rubber can be applied by the use of a pressure spray driven by an electric motor. The author has seen at least one small neat spraying apparatus most suitable for this work and quite inexpensive. Such an apparatus will apply the numerous coats of rubber evenly, quickly and without undue waste.

Drying

The drying of the milk rubber may be speeded up by the use of a hot-air drying oven. A simple Bunsen oven fitted with a thermometer is very suitable. A temperature of about 120° F. will provide the required heat to dry out the latex in a few minutes. Once the cast has become heated in drying out the first coat, succeeding coats will dry out even more rapidly. A more elaborate form of drying oven is a thermostatically-controlled electric hot-air oven. This type of oven will give very accurate control of temperatures, thus avoiding rapid variation in the temperature, with the accompanying risk of damaging the appliances being processed. A drying oven of this type, 14 inches by 18 inches in size, will be adequate for the processing of a number of small appliances at one time. A very satisfactory and inexpensive way of speeding up the drying of individual appliances is a simple process of holding the appliance in front of a gas or electric radiator, care being taken not to scorch the rubber.

Accelerators

Accelerating solutions have been introduced which will induce an instant coagulation of each coat of rubber. By the use of such a medium a succession of coats can be built up in the space of a few minutes, a procedure that would take several hours by natural drying. The accelerators commonly used are acid solutions, the one most used being acetic acid in a strength of 10 to 15 per cent. Other acids which may be used are hydrochloric or sulphuric in 4–8 per cent. strengths. The pad may be dipped into these solutions in a suitable bath or the accelerator may be sprayed on. If dipped, care must be taken that some of the latex does not float off on the surface of the accelerator and re-attach itself to the pad as it is withdrawn from the bath, making the surface rough. If preferred the accelerators can be sprayed on from a squeeze bottle but the spray must be very fine to avoid pitting of the surface.

A disadvantage of acid accelerators is that they tend to form a thin coagulum on the surface of the latex which, being unaffected underneath, still flows freely beneath the surface. A non-acid accelerator, with which this trouble is much reduced, is 10 per cent. of a saturated solution of calcium chloride in water. It appears to make a thicker coagulum and avoids problems of below-surface flow.

Reference has been made in the section on dipping to soaking the cast in a weak acid solution. By this means the accelerator is made to act on the underside of the latex in which the cast is dipped. The real advantage of this is that by suspending the cast in a latex bath for a few minutes a really thick latex coating is built up. The longer it is left immersed the thicker the coat becomes. The cast should be removed when the desired thickness is attained and should be air dried. Dipping in or spraying with accelerator is no advantage as the coat of latex being thick dries more quickly and evenly without a surface coagulum being formed. The 10 per cent. calcium chloride solution is most effective when used in this way.

PROCESSES

As a result of an experiment extending over a number of years the writer has devised, in addition to the purely rubber appliances, two other forms of replaceable shields involving the use of latex milk rubber. Thus three processes are presented for consideration. The first is: appliances made by the coating of a plaster cast with successive layers of milk latex in which padding of suitable materials is introduced. The second is one in which a soft leather is introduced as the foundation of the appliance and upon which the padding and latex coatings are superimposed. The third involves a more complicated processing technique. In this process a soft leather foundation is used with torsion strips and reinforcement of cotton bandage. This appliance may be completed by an outer cover of thin pliable leather. As in the first and second process, padding is introduced at the appropriate stage. The third type of device, although equally soft and resilient on the contact side, is firmer than those previously described and has the great advantage of retaining its shape throughout the whole of its life. This form of appliance, if skilfully made, is by no means bulky, and if suitable leathers are used can be produced with an excellent finish that will delight both the practitioner and patient. The author proposes to describe each type of appliance in detail, with modifications of each for consideration.

PROCESSING OF TYPE I

The advantages of this type of appliance are minimum bulk, resilience, simplicity and speed of processing. The shield can be made entirely of rubber latex and sponge rubber.

The first coats of latex can be applied by dipping, spraying or soaking. For the first two methods the cast may be soaked in water first or receive a prior coat of sealant such as shellac or cellulose cement but experience has shown that the cast can be dipped or sprayed dry quite successfully and that a heavy layer of talcum powder rubbed well into the surface helps subsequent release of the appliance from the cast without impairing coagulation of the latex.

The equipment necessary is a dish of appropriate size to contain the latex, and the dish for the accelerating agent. The cast is first dipped in the latex, gently moved about to ensure a thorough coating (Fig. 38), after which it is withdrawn and the surplus shaken off. It is then held, apex uppermost, to allow the latex to flow back evenly over the cast. After holding it for a few moments in this position, the cast is immersed in the accelerating solution, withdrawn, the excess solution gently shaken off, and the cast again immersed in the latex. This procedure is repeated until four or five coats of the milk rubber have been applied. A sponge rubber pad is cut to shape, bevelled, and the aperture on the underside is also bevelled to ensure that the pad fits snugly against the contour of the prominence which it is designed to protect. According to the desire of the practitioner, the protection may be designed in the form of a crescent pad or an oval shield with aperture. (In the case of appliances necessitating props, these are shaped according to requirements.) The most perfectly shaped pad is produced by fixing it in position, rough-shaping the outside with scissors and finishing this process on a high-speed emery wheel. When completed, the pad is fixed firmly in position with rubber solution. When secured, it is trimmed to conform to the required contour, although the author has found it more satisfactory to complete the shaping of the pad before attaching it. On completing the pad it is covered with rubber solution to seal it before the final coats of latex are applied. After the final dipping in the accelerating agent, the appliance should be immersed in a strong solution of ammonia to neutralise the action of the acid. It is next rinsed thoroughly under running water. Although thorough rinsing in water would remove the acid, it is advisable to make sure that none remains in contact with the rubber by using a neutralising agent (Fig. 39). On completion of processing, the cast is set aside for from twenty-four to forty-eight hours to complete the curing process. The next stage is thoroughly to dust the appliance with talcum powder, carefully to peel it off the cast and to trim off surplus with scissors. A tough and substantial appliance can be produced by the application of ten to twelve coats, although a more delicate appliance, but one which will wear reasonably well, can be produced with a total of eight coats or less.

If the soaking method, which is particularly suitable for making bunion and hallux valgus shields, is used, the cast should first be prepared by immersing it in a 10 per cent. calcium chloride solution or an acid coagulant for about ten minutes. The cast is then dried and immersed in the latex solution and left soaking for anything up to ten or even fifteen minutes to allow a good layer of rubber to build up on the surface.

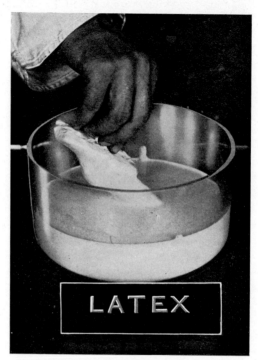

FIG. 38

Dipping the appliance into latex (note apex first).

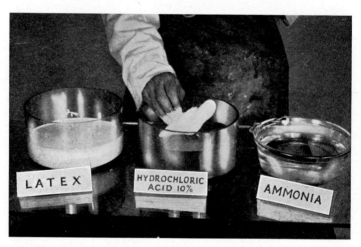

FIG. 39

Appliance leaving the accelerator solution, apex first, to allow the acid to drain back over the cast and drip into the dish.

It should then be removed and air dried. When dry the sponge padding is applied by adhering it with rubber solution. When this is firmly in place, any final trimming or scouring can be done and the surface should be sealed with rubber solution to prevent absorption of liquid latex into the sponge on subsequent immersion. This, if allowed to happen, would harden in the sponge rubber cells and destroy its sponginess.

The appliance is finished by soaking in latex for a few more minutes to give a smooth surface. It should again be dried in air, then powdered with talcum or french chalk, removed from the cast and trimmed to shape. For this process either raw rubber latex may be used or the more sophisticated pre-vulcanised pink latex. Most operators now seem to prefer the latter as it makes a firmer, more durable article of greater patient acceptance.

To assist evaporation of perspiration on wearing, an appropriate number of perforations may be made in the appliance by the use of a leather punch. Patients wearing appliances of this nature should be advised to wash them frequently in warm water to which a little mild non-irritant antiseptic has been added, after which the pad should be thoroughly dusted with an antiseptic powder. An appliance of this nature may be strengthened by reinforcing it with tulle or fine cotton bandage. Where it incorporates the use of a toe glove, a reinforcing strip may be passed round the toe. This strip will prevent longitudinal stretch and possible displacement of the appliance. A reinforcing strip may be applied to the main body of the device, but where a prominence is involved an aperture should be cut in the material to avoid undue pressure on its apex. The reinforcement should be applied after the third or fourth coat. When it is decided that the rubber should not contact the skin, the appliance may be lined with soft leather, e.g. surgical wash-leather. This may be secured either by the use of latex or rubber solution. It is not, however, practical to line deep cavities in this way; for instance, this could not be carried out in a toe glove fitting of an appliance. The author, however, feels that if a leather lining is desired, technique No. 2 or 3 is indicated, as this begins upon a foundation of leather which meets the need in a more satisfactory way. A large variety of appliances can be made by the first process, however, which give great relief to the patient. Whilst the purely rubber appliances made from raw latex have an appreciable life, they do tend to deteriorate, losing their elasticity and shape as a result of body heat and excretion from the skin. When the appliances are reinforced or made with pre-vulcanised latex they retain their shape for a longer period. Devices made by this process have been used successfully for the protection of first and fifth metatarsal bunions and exostoses, chronic corns on the lesser toes, and callosities associated with the hyperextension of the distal joint of the first toe.

As an alternative to sponge rubber, felt padding may be used. In this case the external surface of the pad may be trimmed carefully with scissors or skiving knife and the surface must be sealed with rubber solution before dipping.

Hammer Toe—Shield and Prop

In preparing a toe cast for this type of appliance it is necessary to include a portion of the metatarsus because the appliance is designed with a small tab which lies against the dorsal surface of the metatarsus and is used to pull on the appliance. The chiropodist now makes a crescent pad of surgical sponge. This is used to protect the dorsal aspect of the inter-phalangeal joint. The thickness of the pad is determined by the prominence of the joint or excrescence, usually $\frac{1}{4}$ inch sponge rubber meets the case. When this pad is completed an oblong-shaped pad is made, which is used to fit on the plantar aspect of the joint. This type of pad is termed a plantar prop and acts as a rest for the toe. In the completed appliance not only does the dorsal pad protect the joints from pressure and the plantar prop act as a rest for the toe, but the forward set of the plantar prop induces a lever action in wear, producing a mild corrective effect. When the pad and prop are completed the next step is to apply the preliminary coatings of latex to the cast. This is done in the manner previously described. In dipping the cast in the latex, care should be taken to include the portion of the cast representing the metatarsus. Next the pad and prop are coated with rubber solution, and secured in the respective positions. The pads should be firmly pressed in position to ensure this.

The dipping process is now continued for the further six coats, after which the cast is rinsed in clean water and placed aside for some twenty-four to forty-eight hours to complete curing.

When the rubber is cured, the appliance is liberally dusted with powdered chalk or talcum powder, after which it is carefully peeled off the cast. Having been thoroughly dusted inside and out with the powder, surplus rubber is trimmed off with scissors, the pad being reduced to its final shape. Care should be taken to see that a tab of appropriate size is retained. As previously mentioned, this tab lies against the dorsum and is used to pull the pad into position on the toe. At the discretion of the practitioner, the appliance may be left as a toe glove type, the toe being completely enclosed, or the apex of the appliance may be trimmed off, making it an open-end type of appliance. In either case a suitable number of perforations may be made in the appliance by using a leather punch (Fig. 40).

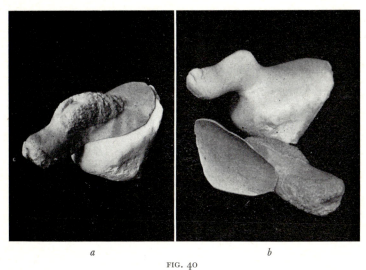

a   *b*

FIG. 40

a. Appliance for terminal and dorsal corn. Type II. *b*. Terminal and dorsal corn. Showing cast and finished shield. Type II.

Appliance for Terminal Corn

This form of appliance is particularly successful and is a means of much comfort to many patients. The sponge rubber for this appliance is shaped in the form of a plantar shaft pad, which extends from the base of the toe along its plantar aspect to the free edge of the nail. The pad widens slightly towards its distal end. A U-shaped cut-out is now made at this end of the pad, which when placed on the appliance is fitted with the shoulders of the 'U' fitting snugly round the site of the excrescence, thus relieving it from pressure. In making this pad the chiropodist should proceed as already described, dipping the pad in the necessary preliminary coats, the fitting of the pad, and resumption of dipping to complete the appliance. Any final shaping of the pad by trimming or scouring should be done before the final coats are applied.

Shield for Fifth Toe

A painful excrescence frequently occurs on the fifth toe as this digit is particularly exposed to pressure and irritation. It is therefore not surprising that this lesion often degenerates into a condition of chronic inflammation, with fibrosis of the tissue. An excrescence of this type lends itself particularly to treatment by replaceable shields. The protective sponge rubber shield for this condition is frequently found most suitable if designed as an oval pad with aperture, although in certain circumstances the crescent-shaped shield proves

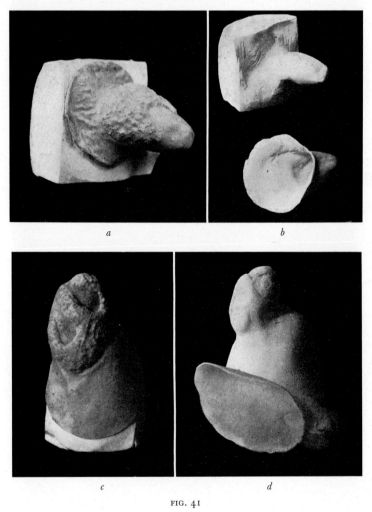

FIG. 41

a. Simple crescent shield for corn on fifth toe. Type II. *b.* Showing cast and shield. Type II. *c.* Double-crescent shield for corns situated on dorsal and lateral aspects of fifth toe. Type II. *d.* Double-crescent shield showing cast and shield. Type II.

suitable. In the case of the oval shield, the aperture should be placed towards the anterior aspect of the shield. Whilst being of sufficient thickness to offer resilient protection, this pad should not be unduly bulky. The margin should be carefully graduated away to blend into the appliance as a whole. The cast for this appliance should extend generously up the lateral border of the foot so as to provide for a substantial tab. The latter is necessary, as when hose are worn the tab is held securely against the foot and the pad firmly secured (Fig. 41, *a* and *b*). When there is an excrescence occurring at the lateral base of the nail and the interphalangeal joint, the pad may be made as a double-crescent shield, the anterior shoulder moulding round the anterior aspect of the first excrescence, the posterior shoulder moulding round the posterior and dorsal aspect of the second excrescence, the central tail extending up between them. In moulding the anterior shoulder of the pad round the excrescence, care should be taken to avoid the nail as far as possible. This pad, like the one previously described, should not be unduly bulky (Fig. 41, *c* and *d*).

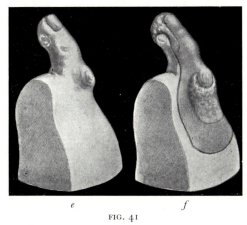

e   f

FIG. 41

e. Cast showing situation of corns. *f*. Finished shield
on cast. Note interdigital pad anterior to corn.

Heloma Molle (Interdigital Fifth)

This device consists of a toe glove appliance with a tab extending well down the lateral border of the foot. The interdigital aspect of the toe glove, however, is cut away up to the anterior margin of the excrescence, the sponge pad being sited on this anterior portion, acting as an interdigital wedge, keeping the toes separated, preventing pressure on the excrescence and allowing free aeration. When corns occur on the interdigital and lateral aspects of the toe, a combination of crescent and wedge may be used (Fig. 41*e* and *f*).

Bunion Shield

One of the most useful latex appliances is the bunion shield, which provides an ideal means of shielding the chronic bunion from friction and pressure. This appliance may be made with toe glove and toe loop. The processes for this appliance are the same as for the appliances previously described and differ little except that it is a larger edition. It will be found advantageous, however, to reinforce the bunion shield with strips of cotton bandage or tulle. In making the pad for this appliance one has the choice between the oval pad with aperture and the crescent-shaped pad. When the aperture or crescent has been cut out, the edge should be bevelled so that when the pad is fitted the angle of the aperture or crescent coincides with the slope of the prominence (Fig. 42*a*). This bevelling enables the pad to be moulded closely to the joint. If the aperture is not bevelled the pad would stand back from the joint, leaving a vertical step which would considerably detract from the pad's effectiveness. When the first four to five coats of latex have been applied to the cast, the pad should be fitted in position and shaped with the scissors to conform roughly to the contours (Fig. 42*b*). If an emery wheel is not available, shaping should be completed with scissors. The emery wheel, however, enables the practitioner to reduce the sponge in a clean and uniform manner so that the completed appliance has a more finished appearance (Fig. 42*c*). When the final trimming of the pad is completed and it is sealed with rubber solution, a piece of the cotton reinforcing material should be cut to the size of the shield and in the shape of a crescent or horse-shoe. The material should now be dipped in latex and applied to the appliance with the tails of the horse-shoe forward. These should be stretched taut round the margins of the pad and brought together at the base of the toe. A strip of reinforcement is now run round the edge of the toe joining up with the reinforcement of the pad. When the reinforcement is pressed firmly into position, dipping is continued until the required number of coats have been applied. The application of the horseshoe-shaped reinforcement at tension round the margin of the pad helps the pad in retaining its shape in wear, whilst the strip round the toe prevents elongation of the toe above, thus the pad cannot be distorted in wear. Curing and trimming are completed as in the pads previously described. This reinforcing process may be equally successfully applied to the lesser pads. Pads so reinforced

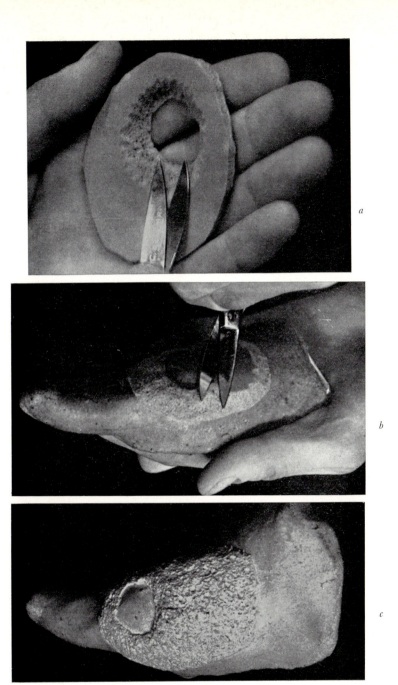

FIG. 42

a. Shaping underside of bunion pad. *b.* Shaping of the surgical sponge on the cast. *c.* Pad scoured to the desired shape.

G

are not so easily damaged or torn and retain their shape longer in wear.

Protective Shield for Calcaneal Exostosis

For this purpose a cast is taken of the heel, care being taken to hold the foot at right angles when the impression is being taken. In making the pad for this appliance it is found that a pear-shaped pad and channel for the tendo Achillis is very suitable. Great care should be taken to shape this pad correctly, the aperture and bevelling should fit accurately to the exostosis. It is a good plan to fit a U-shaped reinforcement completing with a straight strip running round the approximate margin of the appliance, this being applied as a stirrup, the ends being brought together above the pad (see Fig. 43). In moulding this appliance, care should be taken to see that there is sufficient extension beneath the heel to ensure it being secured in position when the stocking is pulled into place.

PROCESSING OF TYPE II

Bunion Shield

The second type of latex appliance differs from the first in that it is built upon a foundation of soft chamois leather or doeskin. In every other respect these appliances are constructed in the same way as the all-rubber type, with the exception of the method of applying the first coat of latex milk rubber. This first coat should be applied very thinly and lightly, so that it does not soak through the leather. When this preliminary coat has been applied, it is advisable to dry it off by applying gentle heat, e.g. holding the cast in front of a gas or electric radiator. Great care should be taken to avoid over-heating or scorching of the appliance. For this first thin coat very little heat is required as the stabiliser will be evaporated and the rubber cured in a comparatively short space of time. When this has been achieved, the process may proceed as in Type I, or the remaining coats may be applied with a brush and the rubber cured by hot air after each application. In this second process the padding is fitted after about three to four coats of the latex milk rubber have been applied. Should the operator desire to complete the process by using an accelerator after the first application of latex he may do so, providing that the first coat is cured by the use of heat. It should be realised that as the accelerator is an acid solution the leather will be seriously damaged should the solution come into contact with it. To avoid this, care should be taken to ensure that the first coat of latex covers the whole of the leather likely to be brought into contact with the acid, as by this precaution the skin of rubber will completely protect the leather. An alternative method of protecting the wash-leather, which has proved highly successful, is to apply a thin, even coat of rubber solution, after which a succession of latex layers can be applied either by the brushing or dipping method. The advantage of the solution method is that if lightly and evenly applied, there is no risk of its soaking through the wash-leather, and a positive protection is provided, leaving the wash-leather lining of the finished appliance unblemished. The method

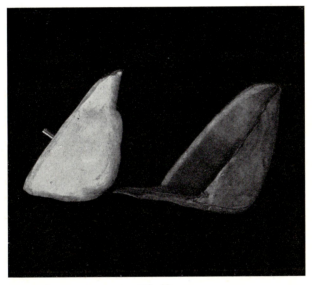

FIG. 43
Protective shield for calcaneal exostosis.
(Note screw inserted in plaster to form a dipping handle.)

of fitting the leather to the cast is one which requires a reasonable combination of care and skill. A very fine textured chamois leather or doeskin should be used, and for lesser toe appliances a very thin leather should be chosen for the purpose. In cutting out the leather it is advisable to place the cast on the skin and then gently lay the leather round it. It should then be held in position while the leather is cut close to the edge of the cast, only a small margin beyond the cast being left. When the leather has been cut out, the portion which fits round the toe of the cast should be stretched and moulded round it so as to leave a surplus at the edges, which is turned back to expose the underside. These exposed surfaces are treated with latex milk rubber or rubber solution, which is brushed on lightly and thinly, after which it is dried off by use of heat as previously described. When this has been accomplished, the edges are nipped firmly together round the toe, which becomes enclosed in a glove finger. The surplus is now trimmed off, the leather being trimmed almost flush to the toe of the cast. Great care, however, must be taken not to burst the edges open. Latex or rubber solution is now brushed over the edges and dried in the manner previously described, after which a strengthening tape made from a strip of cotton bandage or suitable material treated with latex or rubber solution is pressed firmly in position along the edge, securing it to make it firm and strong.

The remaining leather covering the body of the cast is stretched tightly over it so that all the curves and contours are firmly embraced by the material. The leather, as it is stretched over the cast, can be secured by lacing, using a needle and strong linen thread (Fig. 44),

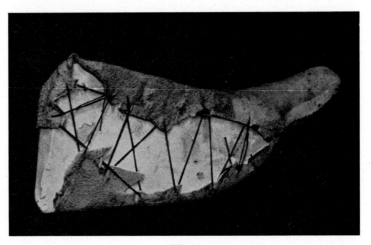

FIG. 44

Method of lacing on the basic leather when a lining is required.

or by tacking with a staple gun (Fig. 45). In lacing the leather into position it is advisable to stretch it over the edges of the cast with the fingers, securing it by stitching it with the needle and thread. Should the chiropodist endeavour to draw the leather over by passing the needle through it and pulling on the thread, he will find the thread will tear through the soft delicate leather. An alternative method of securing the leather is to cut a strip of cotton bandage, apply latex to it, dry it and then cut it into narrow strips about $\frac{1}{8}$ inch wide. The leather is stretched over with the fingers, a little latex applied to the part stretched over, the end of the securing strip of cotton bandage pressed firmly upon it, after which the opposing corner of leather is stretched over it, treated likewise with latex, the strip stretched across and secured to it. It is taken backwards and forwards across the cast in this way until the leather is completely secured. In making small toe casts involving plantar props, the seam can be arranged to come beneath the toe so that it is concealed when the prop is applied. In the case of the bunion shield, the seam can be arranged to occur on the interdigital aspect of the toe. Although the second types of appliances are soft and kind to the skin, they do not keep their shape any longer than those made entirely of rubber. Their advantage lies in having a soft leather as an alternative to the rubber next to the skin.

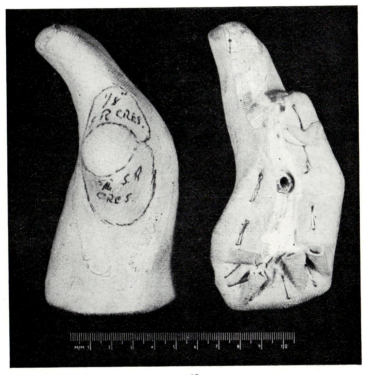

FIG. 45

Chamois leather stretched over cast and held in position by wire staples. Note. Torsion strips and reinforcement to join on inner side of toe. Also hole from which a cup hook has been removed. This hook facilitates handling and hanging up to dry.

PROCESSING OF TYPE III

Bunion Shield

The preparation of this type of appliance is begun in the same way as for Type II, the soft leather base being fitted to the cast in exactly the same manner. The deviation from this type arises following the application of the pad, as it is at this stage that the reinforcing strips are introduced. The strips are made from cotton bandage treated with latex milk rubber. A strip about ½ inch wide is carried from a point just anterior to the joint and at the base of the toe around the margin of the cast, along what would constitute the plantar aspect of the joint, finishing at a point on the middle posterior aspect of the cast or just beyond it. When this torsion strip is applied it should be held taut and kept tightly stretched during its application, its front point of anchorage being firmly secured by the thumb. A similar strip is now applied to the dorsal aspect, this strip slightly overlapping the first (Fig. 46). Two further strips are now applied

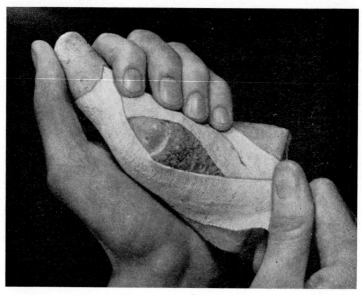

FIG. 46

Applying the torsion strips.

in a similar fashion, partially overlapping the first, but set further back towards the apex of the appliance. A final strip is now applied down the centre of the appliance if desired, thus completely enclosing it in the reinforcing material. This final strip is laid on the appliance and not applied under tension. In this third process a further two coats of latex are all that is necessary to apply after the fitting of the padding and before the application of the torsion strips. When the torsion strips have been applied a further coat is advised. The outer leather, which should be very thin and soft, a fine basil split being very suitable, should be cut to shape by laying on the cast in the

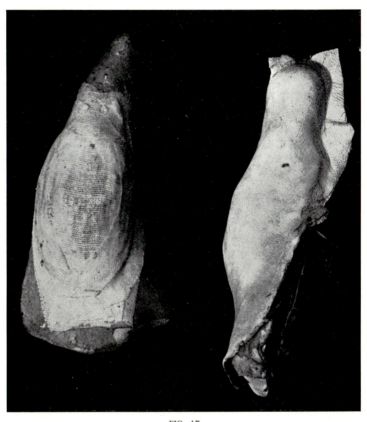

FIG. 47

Torsion strips and laminations completed (*left*). The covering leather stretched over and the edges nipped round the toe (*right*).

same way as for the foundation leather, but a considerably more generous margin should be allowed. The underside of the leather should be treated with latex, which should be dried and the leather applied (Fig. 47), care being taken to avoid as far as possible undue stretching on. Whereas the first leather should be firmly stretched on the cast, this outer cover should only be laid on, because if this is

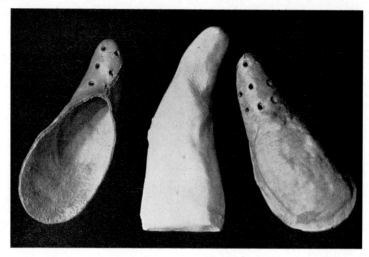

a

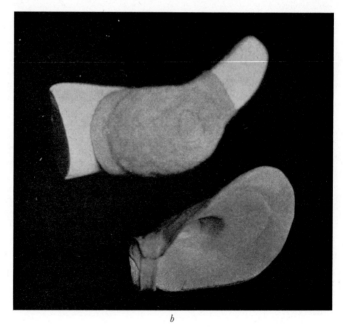

b

FIG. 48

a. Completed bunion shields, toe glove type with inner lining and top
cover. *b*. Toe loop bunion shields. Appliance on the cast shows Type II.
The other is Type III, covered inside and out with basil split.

put on at considerable tension there is a risk of some degree of distortion when the appliance is removed from the cast, owing to contraction of the rubber. Rubber solution may be used as a satisfactory alternative for the attachment of the covering leather. However, if care is taken in applying the outer cover, this appliance will be very firm and will retain its shape throughout the whole of its life. It should be noted that although the appliance is much firmer and stronger than those previously described, the part coming in contact with the skin is just as soft and resilient as those of less robust construction. If thin leathers are used, this type of appliance need not necessarily be more bulky than that of Type I or Type II (Figs 48a and 48b). It should be pointed out, however, that although this method of processing is ideally suited for the larger shields and appliances, it is not suitable for the small appliances for the lesser toes. As an alternative to the toe glove type of bunion shield made by this third process, a toe loop appliance can be made which often pleases the patient who dislikes the feeling of the whole toe being enclosed. In processing, the basil leather is only carried forward of the joint and does not involve the toe. Before fitting the final covering leather, the loop is made, consisting of a strip of chamois leather, which is latexed on one side and folded over, enclosing a tape of cotton material. The latter is to prevent stretch in wear. This loop strip is now placed round the toe to measure the correct length required. It should be long enough for the ends to extend to about $\frac{1}{4}$ inch on the shield. The ends are now bevelled, latex rubber is applied, dried and the loop placed in position round the toe, the ends being firmly pressed in place on the shield. The shield is now finally latexed, as is also the outer cover, which, when dried, is pressed in position. The lacing is now cut and the appliance is slipped off the cast, the loop being passed over the toe, trimming and shaping proceeding in the normal fashion.

In conclusion, it should be mentioned that the bunion shield in Type II can be made into a toe loop appliance by cutting off the glove, leaving only sufficient width to provide a loop round the toe. If desired, this loop can be reinforced by the application of a tape and additional coats of latex.

7

Moccasin Techniques

THE practitioner meets with cases in which some congenital or acquired deformity of the foot so upsets the normal distribution of weightbearing as to cause abnormal pressure areas which are extremely painful. Such cases, when they present themselves for treatment, are of a chronic character. Not infrequently traumatic ulcers result from continuous pressure and irritation over callous formation.

Deformities resulting in lesion of this type arise in cases of spastic paralysis, spina bifida and chronic rheumatic conditions.

Great accuracy in the fitting of any protective device is required, and anything that is liable to become dislodged, even to the slightest degree, will be doomed to failure. It was in an endeavour to overcome this particular problem that the author carried out experimentation with various forms of permanent padding. The outcome of this line of investigation was what is best termed a moccasin appliance, for the simple reason that it is merely a soft moccasin slipper made from chamois leather, surgical sponge and latex rubber. Some degree of body can be given to the upper by using a layer of cotton bandage between the leathers.

To make a device of this nature it is necessary to take a cast of the whole foot, and a deep slipper cast will enable the chiropodist to obtain a positive cast adequate for his requirements. The case sheet should contain the fullest information on the varying degrees of pressure at different points, any peculiarities in angulation, inversion, eversion, hyperextension, etc. This information is essential to enable the chiropodist to make an appliance which will not only relieve pressure from painful areas but will, as far as possible, stabilise the foot in the shoe by general diffusion of weight over the whole plantar area.

As this appliance is made on a plaster cast of the foot, it fits snugly to the tissues, gripping the foot firmly. So accurately does the appliance conform to the foot that this soft, resilient device has repeatedly provided the only solution to many post-operative problems. In cases coming within the aforementioned category, this appliance is made with a lining of fine surgical chamois leather and padded with soft sponge rubber. The outer cover may also be chamois leather or a fine basil split or glove kid. In the case of the amputation of all or any of the appendages, a frontal extension of soft sponge rubber can be fitted to the moccasin and shaped to give a general outline of a perfect foot when a stocking is worn over it (Fig. 49). In doing this the first two or three vertical layers of sponge rubber should be of the soft compression latex foam type in order to cushion the scars of the amputation site and to form a flexible hinge so the dummy toe block can flex on the forefoot stump in walking. The more distal layers of sponge rubber should be of firmer compression in order to prevent the foot slipping forward as well as to support the toe cap of the shoe and maintain its correct outline in wear. The fitting of a forward extension of this nature also enables the forepart of the shoe to be filled. In this way unsightly creases on the vamp of the shoe are prevented, and also a greater degree of stability is achieved. Furthermore, a shoe which looks and feels normal eliminates a tendency to self-consciousness (Fig. 50).

A fine piece of chamois leather is placed over the plantar surface of the cast, bringing it over the back of the heel up to the required depth and over the ends of the toes on to the dorsum of the foot. The leather is now brought up the side of the foot, which will result in the formation of a pleat at each corner. The pleats should be cut away and the inner edges latexed. When these are dry, they should be nipped together (Fig. 51), trimmed flush and secured with tapes of cotton bandage. In this way the foundation of the moccasin has been created. When nipping the edges together, care should be taken to see that the moccasin fits tightly on to the cast, particularly round the upper margin. The next stage in this process is to coat the whole moccasin with latex and allow to dry. Drying, of course, can be accelerated if the cast is held in front of a radiator. Care, however, should be taken to avoid scorching. In applying this first coat a soft brush should be used and the latex coating applied very lightly and thinly.

This somewhat light and delicate method of applying the latex is necessary to avoid it soaking through the chamois leather to the inside and spoiling, to some extent, the effect and appearance of the inner lining. Two or three further coats may now be applied liberally, as, providing the first coat is thoroughly dry, it is not possible for the liquid to soak through, the first coat having formed a thin protective

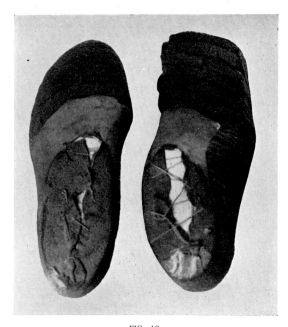

FIG. 49

(*Right*) Latex foam built onto the forepart of the moccasin prior to the final shaping. (*Left*) Foam extension scoured to shape.

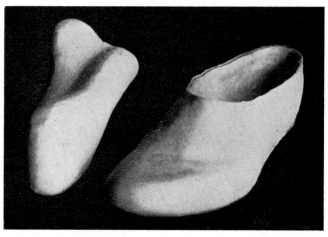

FIG. 50

The cast and the completed false toe moccasin.

skin. When the final coat of latex thoroughly dries, the practitioner should prepare the surgical sponge protective padding. This soft resilient material should fit very close round the various prominences, constituting pressure points. Padding should also be applied to the concavity of the long arch, the object of the padding being not only to remove pressure from the painful areas by padding round them but to apply the padding in such a way as to diffuse the pressure over the whole plantar area. The chiropodist should, as far as possible, aim at stabilising the foot in the shoe and, as a consequence, some degree of wedging may be necessary. The padding should be just adequate to relieve pressure and no more, and should be trimmed

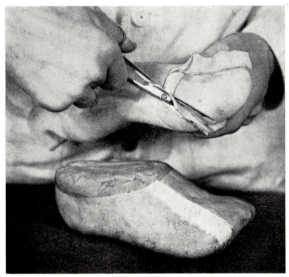

FIG. 51

Trimming the seam flush prior to taping. The taped seam can be clearly seen on the cast in the foreground.

in such a way as to leave a clean uniform under-surface. The insulation is completed by a final sole of thin sponge fitted over the whole plantar area. It is usually found advisable to reinforce the wash-leather constituting the upper of the moccasin to prevent its becoming stretched and mis-shapen in use. This is done by applying one or two layers of cotton bandage which have, as previously described, been treated with latex. The moccasin is now ready for the final cover, which can be also of chamois leather or of very fine basil split, which presents a smooth, soft surface not so easily soiled as the former leather. The outer cover should be cut generously and applied in the same manner as the first leather cover, except that whilst the former is stretched tightly on to the cast, this should be laid gently over the appliance and not stretched on. The reason for this is that when it is stretched on it will tend to contract when the appliance is removed from the cast and so distort it. The only part where stretching-on is advisable in this outer cover is at the point representing the actual upper margin of the cover. The edges which have been nipped together at the four corners can be trimmed flush with a pair of scissors and will remain perfectly secure. The joints will be very neat in appearance (Fig. 52).

The moccasin is now gently removed from the cast; this will be somewhat difficult as the moccasin will naturally be a tight fit. After it has been removed, however, the upper margin of the appliance can be trimmed and shaped.

Golosh Type Upper

The outer cover may be cut as a U-shaped piece to fit over the front of the cast and along the sides. When this has been moulded on and the ends nipped together at the back, it should be moulded on to the plantar surface and the surplus skived away.

The appliance is completed by fitting a sole of a more substantial leather, sheepskin being very suitable. The finished appliance resembles a slipper with a golosh upper (Fig. 53).

The moccasin appliance can also be processed by the dipping method, using an accelerator. When using this technique it is advisable to seal the top edges of the leather with adhesive tape so as to prevent the latex milk rubber from finding its way between the leather and the cast and thus spoiling the lining. As in the case of other latex shields in which the dipping method is used, a coating of rubber solution should be applied to the leather before dipping is commenced. Three to four coats of latex should be applied before the padding is placed in position, after which a further three or four coats will complete the appliance with the exception of the outer leather. If the appliance is to be worn in a strong shoe, it can be strengthened by additional coats of latex. The secret of success in this type of appliance is to provide just the right degree of resilient support to prevent impingement upon the pressure areas whilst at the same time providing a slight amount of general insulation, achieving this combination with a minimum of bulk.

Moccasin appliances can be modified in many ways to meet individual cases; in their application the practitioner will find ample scope for his ingenuity.

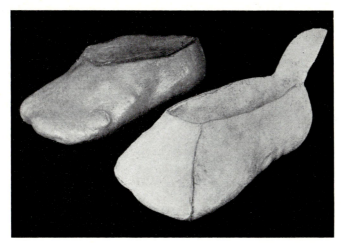

FIG. 52

Finished moccasin appliance, non-golosh type.

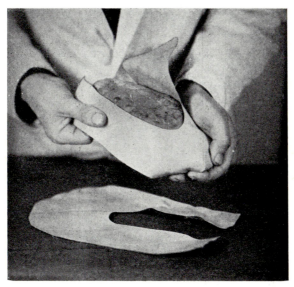

FIG. 53

Fitting of the golosh type outer leather to a moccasin appliance.

The author has found that in some cases where the moccasin is designed for the protection of lesions or painful areas on the plantar aspect only, it is an advantage to cut away the upper over the toes, leaving only a collar round the instep. The modification makes the appliance much less bulky in the forepart, whilst the combination of the collar round the top ensures that it is retained securely in position on the foot.

Another improvement is to make numerous perforations in the upper. These holes should be made with a leather punch, and should be so numerous as to give an openwork basket effect. The aeration of the foot will be greatly improved by this procedure. In some cases it has been found necessary to make an aperture for the great toe; several moccasins of this type have been successfully fitted. In some cases the incorporation of dorsal padding has been successfully carried out. In several cases a tab was fitted at the back of the appliance to assist in pulling it on the foot.

The author has numerous cases on record in which this type of appliance has been the means of solving a long-standing problem. Some examples have been selected and included in this volume, with appropriate clinical photographs (Figs 115, 116, 124, 125, 127, 128, 143, and 146).

The Lace-up Moccasin

To facilitate the putting on and taking off of these moccasins it is sometimes an advantage to make a slit down the front and insert two or three eyelets on either side of the slit so that it may be laced on. A chamois leather tongue should be inserted behind the lace-up to protect the dorsum of the foot.

The Elastic Top Moccasin

An alternative method whereby the moccasin can be made to fit the foot closely yet be capable of easy removal is for a piece of surgical elastic to be inserted all round the top between the inner lining leather and the outer cover. Since the overall depth of the moccasin cannot be increased without its showing above the shoe, the elastic forms the top $\frac{1}{2}$ inch of the upper of the appliance which has to be reduced accordingly.

The method for doing this is as follows. The elastic, usually a 2 inch wide piece of pink elastic net folded to half width, is placed around the moccasin, with the folded edge to the top immediately before applying the final covering of chamois leather. The centre of the folded strip of elastic net is placed at the back of the heel and the two ends are brought forward and stapled down over the dorsum of the forefoot at an angle to each other and under firm tension. The upper and lower edges of the elastic are then marked all round the appliance with a ball-point pen. The elastic is then lifted clear of these marks but the stapled front is not disturbed. A third line is then sketched in midway between the two lines already drawn. Rubber solution is then applied to the lower half and to the corresponding part of the elastic on its inner surface. When tacky the elastic is carefully replaced in position so that only the lower half is adhering to the appliance and the upper half is free. When dry the staples in the front part are removed and the ends are stuck down under tension. The staples are then replaced to hold the tension until the rubber solution is dry when they should be removed before applying the golosh upper. This is now cemented down in position with its upper edge lying along the centre of the elastic net. After cementing the golosh upper over the entire surface of the moccasin and turning the bottom edges onto the sole of the appliance and cementing a sole in place, the elastic is turned back to reveal the ball-point line sketched midway between the upper and lower limits of the elastic. A sharp knife is now introduced to cut through the lining leather all round the cast. The moccasin can now be slipped off the cast and the elastic will be found to be neatly inserted between the inner lining and outer covering leathers all around the top edge.

THE SPLINT BOOT

The splint boot appliance is made on a lower limb cast which extends as high as required to provide adequate support (Figs 135 and 137).

In the case of the post-polio patient with a talipes varus deformity, there is a considerable stress on the ankle joint, particularly involving the outer malleolus and the external lateral ligaments. A marked supination of the foot, usual in this deformity, causes most of the thrust to be taken on the outer border of the foot with the cuboid becoming a painful pressure area. Not only is there much stress and distortion of the outer malleolus, but this area is subjected to much pressure and friction.

The extremely poor circulation and consequential debilitated state of the tissues inevitably results in trophic ulceration. I have seen the whole lateral border of the foot affected from the cuboid to the end of the fifth toe in a chronic state of ulceration as the result of this deformity and a similar state of trophic ulceration of the ankle joint from the wearing of a caliper. It would appear that the usual combination of the surgical boot and caliper was not the answer in these cases.

It is not difficult to find the reason. Stiffening of the boot upper and an extended and strengthened counter, even when some degree of padding was used, did not prevent movement between the foot and the boot when the patient attempted to walk. It is this movement between the supporting structures and the foot that is the basis of failure in the treatment of these cases and I became firmly convinced that only by solving this problem of friction and pressure between the foot and the supporting structures would any progress be made.

After much thought and experiment I devised what is now known as the splint boot, a name I gave the device owing to the fact that it is in the form of a boot in its general appearance, with the foot exposed over the vamp and toe area, although as mentioned later the appliance was originally intended for a spastic case and modified for the talipes varus deformity.

After preliminary treatment of the ulcerated areas, the cast is taken and the boot made on it. A soft chamois leather lining is moulded on to the cast and the lateral surface covered with a soft padding of latex foam rubber. The ulcerated areas are further padded by a layer of firmer textured rubberzote. In this way the tissues are first received by the soft gentle cushioning of the foam rubber and the real protection provided by the firmer material underlying it round the area of the lesions. I next applied lightweight splintage. This very strong feather-weight material, comprising several layers of bandage and cellulose adhesive lamination, is faithfully moulded on the appliance over the padding, the splintage extending from just below the top of the leg over the whole lateral area and extending round the lateral border of the foot onto the sole.

The bottom of the appliance forms a complete sole extending to the end of the toes. The front of the leg is then opened up and eyelets are fitted so that the appliance can be laced and a chamois leather tongue is fitted. It is finished off with a soft outer cover of glove kid or basil leather.

A surgical boot is now made with a cork to stabilise the angulated sole with the floor of the boot. Stability is further assisted by fitting the surgical boot with a floated heel extending forward to fill in the waist in the outer side.

This combination works on the following lines: the splint boot is laced firmly onto the foot to which it is accurately moulded so that no movement can take place. The surgical boot is put on over this and laced firmly on. The padding protects the ulcerated areas which in the absence of movement are not irritated by friction. The splintage gives complete support to the ankle and takes much of the thrust. On walking any friction and pressure by the boot is taken by the splintage, also pressure by the caliper on the outer malleolus is taken on the splintage which provides complete protection to the affected areas. The strength of the splintage is derived from the special combination of materials, cotton bandage and cellulose adhesive laminations invented by the author, and by the fact that it is moulded.

The fact that the splintage and padding are perfectly moulded over the tissues completely diffuses the pressure.

The principle in this technique is to marry the appliance to the limb and so prevent friction when walking by movement between the appliance and the foot. By moulding the padding and the splintage accurately to the contours, pressure is diffused. The strong ultra-lightweight material gains additional strength by the fact that it is moulded and curved around the limb.

The surgical boot is so designed as to stabilise the appliance on a graded cork if necessary. The appliance is assisted in taking the mal-thrust by the floated and extended heel.

This solution to the problem has proved completely successful. In several cases ulceration of long standing cleared up in the matter of a few weeks and the areas remained healed. The combination of the supporting splintage and accommodating surgical footwear gave stability and support, enabling patients who had become completely incapacitated to be mobile again, resume a reasonably active life and again undertake employment.

8

Corrective Surgical Insoles

IN giving consideration to defects of the longitudinal arch it would be as well to contemplate briefly the structure and function of the feet, with special consideration of the arches. If a pedograph is taken of a patient standing with the feet parallel, the footprints show only the heels, the metatarso-phalangeal areas, and the lateral borders. The medial borders of the prints appear concave because the inner longitudinal arches are not in contact with the ground. Ellis informs us that the legs and feet do not constitute two separate pillars, but are two halves of a divided pedestal, each being complementary to the other. When standing we are supported on the outer rim of a more or less complete circle. This outer rim provides the static support, and the raised, domed inner portion forms the lever. This strong resilient arch provides the base from which the body is propelled, whilst the outer rim provides a stable area of support. In 1938, when dealing with this subject, Lambrinudi stated, 'the outer part lies flat on the ground, giving a big weightbearing surface and providing stability and balance with the aid of the fourth and fifth toes. It is essentially a balancing organ, whereas the inner portion is essentially a lever.'

If the leg and foot were stripped of its soft structures down to the ligaments, it would be seen that the foot is not only arched longitudinally, but that there is also a deep transverse arch, making a deep depression running from the anterior border of the calcaneum to the heads of the metatarsals. This transverse arch is deepest under the cuneiforms and cuboid bones. Bridging this from side to side are the strong tendon slips of the insertions of tibialis posticus and peroneus longus, the former running from the inner side and the latter from the outer side. Whilst these are intact the transverse arch cannot be flattened. This is particularly applicable to the peroneus longus, which assists materially in maintaining the transverse arch by pulling the internal cuneiform and first metatarsal towards the cuboid. Whilst the transverse arch is maintained in this manner it is impossible to collapse the long arch. The muscles running from the leg to the foot provide the active support of the arches. They act as slings on each side of the foot, holding up the centre of the long arch. The peroneus longus does this on the outer side and the tibialis posticus on the inner side. They are further assisted in this function by the flexor hallucis longus, which passes along the sole of the foot like a bowstring, and also by the flexor digitorum longus, which passes forward along the plantar surface of the foot.

When considering the bone structure of the arches of the foot they should not be contemplated as an architectural arch locked by a keystone at the summit but as a series of segments arranged in the form of a concavity retained in their relative positions by strong bands of fibrous tissue. These allow limited movement at the articulations and provide an appreciable degree of flexibility in the foot as a whole. The passive support of the arches of the foot is brought about by the peculiar shape of the bones and the strong ligamentous bands which retain them in position, while the active support is provided by the muscles. These give that controlled resilience found in healthy feet. Thus the feet are designed to provide shock absorption and leverage for propulsion.

WEIGHT DISTRIBUTION

When a person with normal legs and feet stands in an erect position, body weight is transmitted in definite proportions to the base of the calcaneum and the heads of the metatarsals. By means of the staticometer, Morton demonstrated that the weight was distributed half to the calcaneum and half to the metatarsals, where the first metatarsal accepts twice the load of the remaining four. It should also be noted that the second, third and fourth metatarsal heads depress on weightbearing taking their proportionate share of the load. The lateral arch is similarly depressed, forming the outer border of the foot into the static buttress or outer rim of the pedestal as described by Ellis and Lambrinudi. The long and short plantar ligaments reinforce and control the lateral segments of the foot, ensuring its stability.

The medial arch, which constitutes the highest part of the concavity of the long arch, is designed to provide some degree of flexibility. It should be understood, however, that the range of depression is limited by the ligaments controlling the bones and is only sufficient to provide the necessary shock absorption. That this restricted degree of depression of the medial arch does take place has been fully demonstrated by the radiologist. At a lecture given in December 1948 by Dr R. G. Ollerenshaw, two radiographs of a normal foot were shown, one non-weightbearing and the other weightbearing. Lines marked at the anterior and posterior extremities of the foot showed that on weightbearing the arch was slightly depressed and the foot lengthened appreciably. The degree of depression of this medial arch in the sound foot is not sufficient to affect the normal stability, since, when the natural limit of movement is reached, the ligaments prevent further depression, and the foot under static pressure becomes a rigid structure with well-balanced weight distribution.

STRUCTURAL AND POSTURAL STABILITY OF THE FOOT

The structural stability of the foot is provided by the bony architecture of the foot as previously outlined, maintained by the peculiar shape of the bones retained in their compact formation by binding ligaments. The postural stability is maintained by a combination of the action of the intrinsic muscles of the foot and the muscles of the leg, which maintain a constant balance of the tibia in relation to the talus, and thus body weight is transmitted in correct proportions to the bearing surfaces of the foot. This is ensured by the muscle tonus and the balanced action of antagonistic muscle groups. Thus we have a stable, rigid base provided by the bony architecture, and postural balance by muscular control.

FACTORS AFFECTING THE STABILITY OF THE FOOT

The stability of the foot may be undermined by defects in the bony architecture, which may be congenital or the result of disease or trauma.

Some Congenital Defects in the Bony Architecture

Developmental defects in one or more bones of the foot may seriously upset its normal architecture, resulting in malfunction and instability.

Short First Metatarsal

This was first stressed by Morton, who stated that a short first metatarsal bone causes the second to act as the principal leverage member. The stresses converge upon the base of the second metatarsal and are transmitted by it to the ground. He goes on to inform us that under the increased amount of function the shaft of the second metatarsal becomes widened and hypertrophied. The effects here are threefold. First, a postural fault will arise owing to the tilting inwards of the medial arch until the head of the first metatarsal becomes weightbearing. This upsets weight distribution through the foot, and undermines the normal triangle of stability. Ligaments are strained and a process of pronation of the foot results. Secondly, the abnormal weightbearing of the second metatarsal will result in weakness of the anterior metatarsal region, causing a dorsal subluxation of the second metatarso-phalangeal joint, with painful callosity under the head of the metatarsal. Thirdly, there may be a traumatic synovitis of the second metatarso-cuneiform joint as a result of strain and irritation.

Hypermobile First Metatarsal

In this condition, which may be congenital or acquired, the stability of the foot will be affected by the elevation of the head of the first metatarsal on weightbearing. This has an effect similar to that of a short first metatarsal, resulting in a falling over inwards of the medial arch. A factor which should also be considered is not essentially an elevation of the head of the metatarsal, but rather a depression of the base in association with a weakness of the retaining structures of the first metatarso-cuneiform articulation.

Metatarsus Primus Varus

This is a further weakness of the architectural structure in which the first metatarsal is deviated medially at an abnormal angle. There is usually also a marked widening of the articulation between the first and second cuneiforms. Weakness of the ligaments is usually associated with metatarsus primus varus, producing the condition of hypermobility of the first metatarsal segment with the inevitable undermining of stability and the clinical feature of some degree of pronation.

Other osseous factors are knock-knee and bow-leg, either of which cause a mal-direction of thrust through the leg onto the foot, upsetting the normal weight distribution.

It will be noted that in all architectural defects ligamentous strain and weakness is inevitable.

Os Tibialis Externum

This is a separate ossification of the tuberosity of the navicular. According to Lake, this structural defect occurs in 10 per cent. or

12 per cent. of people, and causes weak and painful feet. In this condition the inferior calcaneo-navicular ligament may well be involved, and as a result of the weakening of the attachment of this ligament, posture and balance may be affected, involving the medial arch.

Muscular and Ligamentous Strain

Whilst the defects in the osseous structure of the foot almost inevitably undermine the stability of the foot, it should be realised that weakness of ligaments and muscles will affect the stability of a foot even though it is perfect in its bony architecture. The support of the dynamic foot is vested in the muscles, and if these are healthy a degree of contractility is always present, even when the foot is at rest. This degree of contractility is known as muscle tonus. Should the muscles be weakened by illness or disease, muscle tonus will be lost, their function as supports will be impaired, and in proportion to the degree they are affected, strain will be placed upon the ligaments. Continued passive strain on the ligaments will result in their becoming gradually stretched, allowing a range of movement at the joints beyond normal. Thus weakness of muscles will impair postural stability.

Summary. The factors responsible for the maintenance of a healthy foot are a perfect architectural structure with the arrangement of bones well secured by the ligaments and actively supported by muscles. These provide a firm outer buttress, a resilient medial arch and lever, with correct distribution of weight ensuring structural and postural stability in both the static and dynamic foot.

Congenital defects in the osseous architecture of the foot and leg, or muscular weakness, will ultimately affect the stability and function of the foot. Whilst in a number of cases defects in the bony structures of the leg and foot are responsible for postural instability with varying degree of flattened or pronated foot, by far the greater proportion are acquired as the result of external influences. These include such factors as general debility as a result of illness which may or may not confine the patient to bed for a long time, passive strain as the result of long periods of standing in one position, e.g. shop assistants, excessive weightbearing, people carrying heavy loads, pregnancy. Anæmia in a child during the growing period often results in flabby, undernourished muscles which are not able to perform adequately their duty of providing active support for the arches. The patient confined to bed suffers from atrophic muscles which are not able to provide the necessary support when he is up and about again. In the case of the shop assistant, continued passive strain results in muscular fatigue or atonia (loss of muscle tonus), whilst the person carrying heavy weights taxes the muscles beyond their normal capacity, inducing muscle fatigue and atrophy.

FLATTENING AND PRONATION
OF THE FOOT

Pronated Foot

The effect on the postural stability of the foot in the case of a short first metatarsal and a hypermobile first metatarsal have already been mentioned. The foot falls over inwards until the head of the first metatarsal becomes weightbearing. In such cases the tarsus does not flatten, but topples inwards as a unit (Fig. 54). The effect of

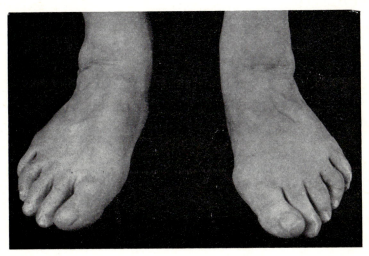

FIG. 54
Mobile pronated feet of a young adult.

this is to place an abnormal strain on the inner capsule of the ankle joint and the internal lateral ligaments. A radiograph (posterior view) of such a case will show eversion of the calcaneum in relation to the tibia, the extent being related to the degree of pronation. The tuberosity of the navicular will also be noted to be very prominent. In the case of the hypermobile first metatarsal and metatarsus primus varus, the shaft of this bone will be shown parallel to the ground. If the patient were to stand on a table with his back to the practitioner it will be noted that the foot will be everted, a marked bulge in the region of the navicular will be observed, and the tendo Achillis will show an inward swerve. Another factor is the plantar flexion of the great toe, caused by an endeavour to regain the stability which has been lost as a result of the hypermobile or short first metatarsal. In the completely pronated foot the lateral border is no longer weightbearing and will be raised.

Contra-Lateral Wedging

In 1946 Mr W. Sayle-Creer, F.R.C.S., stated, 'most cases are not flattened, i.e. badly shaped feet, but are everted, valgus, over-balanced or pronated feet, i.e. feet whose posture is wrong. The treatment required is to restore the posture or balance rather than a hypothetically dropped arch.' He also informs us that in this pronated foot the great toe acts as if it were taking over the support of the inner border of the foot because the first metatarsal is incapable. 'You will often see an over-acting anterior tibial muscle tendon standing out too clearly (which only shows that the trouble is not primarily due to a weak anterior tibial muscle).' A test was then suggested in which the heel is grasped from the back with the thumb on the inner side and the index finger on the outside. The heel is gently but firmly pressed into slight inversion, when the medial arch will be restored. This experiment should always be carried out with a moderately relaxed foot.

Treatment of Pronated Foot

In 1937, in the *Journal* of the British Association of Chiropodists, Mr Sayle-Creer described how he arrived at his own particular method of treating pronated feet by the use of outside sole wedges. He states that as a house surgeon to an orthopædic department 'it fell to my lot to see both severe mobile and rigid forms of flat foot manipulated and put up in plaster of paris. I was taught to invert the heel and apply the plaster on the leg and heel in this position. As soon as this portion was set hard we "untwisted" the forefoot, that is, we everted the forefoot and completed the plaster on what was now a beautifully shaped foot with a good longitudinal arch. This set me thinking, until I realised that if the severe cases needed an everted forefoot so must the simple case, so from then on I discarded the inner sole wedge (Thomas wedge) and either left the sole level or else wedged the outer side.' In the case of the hyper-mobile first metatarsal, it is advisable in carrying out the experiment for reforming the long arch not only to invert the heel but to depress the head of the first metatarsal. In clinical practice the inside of the heel is wedged to hold the heel upright or slightly inverted. This wedge prevents the heel from sagging into eversion. The outside sole wedge assists in everting the forefoot and depressing the head of the first metatarsal. It should be noted that after wedging, the plane or level of the road surface is altered. As a result the shoe will wobble when placed on a flat surface because the wedging of the shoe has caused it to be twisted. It should therefore be untwisted until it stands firmly. The degree of wedging must be determined in each individual case. It is also necessary to watch the reaction after wedging and make modifications accordingly.

The writer carried out this method of wedging over a number of years. This was done in conjunction with progressive remedial exercises, and proved to be a great advance on corrective measures previously used. In the course of clinical observations over a considerable period of time it was noted that in many of the cases the loose fitting of the shoe heel allowed the heel to sag into eversion despite the heel wedge. It was also realised that the considerable variation in wedge thicknesses required resulted frequently in a system of trial and error, necessitating a series of shoe alterations which caused much inconvenience by repeated visits to the shoemaker. I felt, therefore, that the interpretation of this excellent system of correction in a form that would eliminate these defects was very desirable. Such an appliance would be required to hold the foot firmly in the corrected position. When reflecting on the variety of foot types and the varying degrees of elevation of the medial arch, I realised that the appliance must reform each foot to its own natural contours. The device should hold the foot firmly but comfortably in the corrected position and be light, resilient and strong, with a reasonable degree of serviceability.

Flattened Foot

In addition to the pronated foot arising from some architectural defect in the osseous structures, or instability of the first metatarsal segment, a proportion of flattened feet are met with on which a general sagging of the arch structures has taken place. In severe cases of this flaccid type of flattened foot the neck of the calcaneum will be depressed to a marked degree and an obvious gap will be noted in the calcaneocuboid articulation. This flattened foot is met with in cases where the supporting muscles have been very considerably weakened by some serious illness. The writer has seen a number of cases during the examination of the feet of adolescent school children. In such cases the general physique was poor, with muscles underdeveloped and flabby. As in the case of pronated foot, intermediate stages of the condition will be seen. There will also be cases in which a combination of some degree of flattening and pronation occurs. This flattening out of the bony arch is the result of continued strain on the passive supporting structures which are unaided by debilitated muscles. The corrective appliance for either the flaccid flattened foot or the pronated foot aims at reforming the foot into its normal contours. This is achieved in the former case by supporting the bones of the foot and holding them in correct relationship to each other, and in the latter by inverting the heel and everting the forefoot, thus reforming the long arch. In either case the re-establishment of the normal bony architecture of the foot results in a regaining of correct weight distribution and structural stability. Postural stability will eventually be established when remedial exercises and the exercise resulting from use in its corrected position have succeeded in developing muscle tonus and balance in the foot and leg. On reflection, it will be realised that in achieving such an appliance the important factors are design and materials.

In view of the characteristic individuality of feet, it was obvious that the only sound basis from which to start was with a cast of the corrected foot. Casting for this purpose by the negative and positive plaster method was neither convenient nor practical.

Slipper Casting for Correction

Slipper casting was found to be reasonably suitable. These casts can be taken as advocated by Nelson, the patient lying face downwards on a plinth with the legs supported in a semi-flexed position. Nelson claims that the mobile pronated foot regains its normal contours in that position. The casts can be taken, however, quite successfully by sitting the patient in a chiropody chair. The limb should be supported in a semi-flexed position by an assistant. When the plaster bandage has been applied, the foot should be remoulded into a corrected position by inverting the heel, everting the forefoot and at the same time depressing the head of the first metatarsal. It is advisable to press a flat surface gently against the plantar surface of the heel, otherwise the impression of the non-weightbearing heel will not be found suitable in the finished surgical insole.

CORRECTION OF MOBILE PRONATED FOOT BY LAMINATED SURGICAL INSOLES

The writer claims that after numerous experiments he succeeded in designing an appliance which conformed to all the requirements both in its ability to reform the foot and maintain it in correction. It also combines lightness and resilience with strength. The appliance is an insole designed with a cupped heel which extends upwards on the lateral side of the calcaneum as a flange which is reinforced to form a strong buttress. On the medial side a conventional flange extends to beyond the navicular where it is swept in to follow the shaft of the first metatarsal. Returning to the lateral side, it should be noted that this extends as a shallow flange along the lateral border, tapering away almost to nothing behind the head of the fifth metatarsal. The appliance extends to the conventional length of the ordinary arch support, its anterior margin ending just posterior to the heads of the first and fifth metatarsals.

The principle upon which the insole works is as follows: As the insole has been made upon a cast of the corrected foot, the foot when placed upon the appliance must reform to the corrected contours. The heel is guided into its proper seating in the cupped heel by the lateral flange which retains the heel firmly in position. The flange is strongly reinforced, particularly at its outer base, to enable it to resist the thrust of the calcaneum as the foot bears down upon the anterior platform of the appliance. The medial flange, the twist of the plane of the upper surface of the insole and the extension of the lateral flange correct the forefoot. In this way the body-weight acts as a corrective medium as it is transmitted through the weightbearing foot, which is reformed. If the cast of the corrected foot is held on a level with the eyes, plantar surface uppermost and with the heel to the rear, it will soon be seen that the inversion of the heel has resulted in it being on a different plane to the anterior weightbearing surface (the ball of the foot). The plantar surface of the heel inclines upwards to the lateral side, as a result of which an insole made to the cast without some adjustment could not be stabilised in the shoe. It is necessary, therefore, to build up the medial side until a horizontal plane corresponding to the anterior-bearing surface is achieved. An appliance so wedged will be found to stand firm and stable on a flat surface (Figs 55 and 56).

There are some people who dispute that these laminated insoles are corrective. It is necessary to appreciate that the word corrective

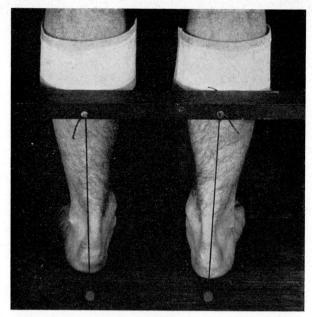

FIG. 55

Plumb-line device showing the swerve of the Achilles tendon in
pronated feet.

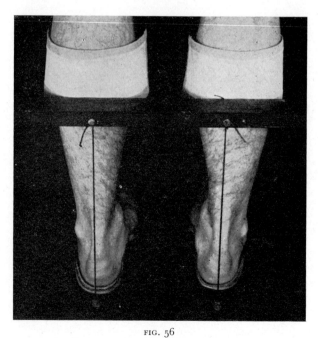

FIG. 56

This plumb-line device clearly shows the corrective effect of the
appliances independent of footwear.

is applied here to position. It is not meant to imply that these insoles are curative.

Strange to relate, however, it has been found in practice that if a series of corrective insoles are made over several years and the amount of correction applied to the foot as each succeeding impression is taken is progressively reduced, there comes a time when the appliances can be dispensed with altogether without a return of symptoms.

This is a process which must not be hurried and is best suited to the treatment of adolescents. When the appliances are finally dispensed with, it is sometimes advisable to continue treatment with medial heel wedges, either with or without the addition of a lateral sole wedge for some time. There is no doubt that, by carefully timed and progressive reduction of the amount of correction applied, it is possible to get the muscles and ligaments restored to their correct function so that no further help is needed.

Materials

The materials used for corrective insoles comprise a natural finish sheepskin which, when dampened, can be stretched over the cast and moulded to every protuberance and depression, cellulose acetate cement of the kind used extensively in the shoe industry, white open-weave cotton bandage and jute scrim. These last two are used for making laminations where a loosely woven cellular material which will hold the cellulose acetate in its cellular spaces is needed. It is useful to have a supply of the cellulose thinner both for thinning the cement and for washing out the brushes with which the cement is applied. Bottom filler compound, consisting of granulated cork with cellulose acetate cement, again a shoe industry material, is useful to fill up hollows and to square off a cupped heel seat. It has, however, little intrinsic strength and needs to be used mixed with an equal volume of cellulose acetate cement to prevent its crumbling in wear and is now little used in this work.

Leather is used for the final coverings. Usually a thin natural light-coloured basil or a thin grain split is used on the surface which comes against the foot and a darker and heavier leather, usually a basil, on the outer surface which comes in contact with the shoe. (The subject of leather and its use in chiropodial orthopædics is discussed more fully in the last section of Chapter 15.)

A further development of corrective surgical insole making involves the use of heat-softening polythene sheet. The one preferred is Vitrithene which is flesh coloured and translucent and is supplied in sheets 36 inches square. The ⅛ inch thick sheet is preferred for this work. A piece of the plastic is cut large enough to cover the required area of a plaster cast. The cast is turned sole up and the piece of plastic is laid on it. Both are then heated in an oven or under a grill until the plastic loses its translucency and becomes transparent. Care should be taken not to allow heating to continue beyond this point or the plastic will become partly fluid and distortion of the final appliance will occur.

On removal from the heat the plastic is pressed down onto the cast with a well gloved hand and moulded to the shape of the cast. On cooling it hardens and is cut or scoured to shape. This results in a very strong and durable inlay.

The same material and method can be employed in the making of a rigid splint boot (Chapter 7). The warmed plastic sheet can be moulded over a cast from the metatarsal heads to well above the ankle. A second heating may be needed to close the plastic over the dorsum and up the front of the leg as well as to ensure a close fit around heel and ankles. The splint boot can be sprung off the cast in the same way as it is sprung onto and off the patient's foot and ankle. A tongue and eyelets can be fitted and padding can be adhered inside if required.

LAMINATED SURGICAL INSOLES

The laminated insole technique was devised to enable the appliances to be moulded on a cast of the foot without involving the use of complicated and expensive apparatus. By the method devised by the author, insoles can be made that will fit accurately to the contours of the foot thus diffusing weightbearing pressure and providing stability.

In the case of corrective surgical insoles, the appliance secures the foot in the corrected position (Fig. 66, *top left*).

Leathering

The appliances are made on a base of soft basil or other suitable leather which is stretched over the cast. The leather is cut to a size and shape that will adequately cover the plantar surface of the cast and extend well up the sides and round the heel. The leather is then wetted so that it can be stretched over the contours of the cast. It should not be soaked but adequately moistened.

The leather may be attached in any of three ways, namely lacing (Fig. 57), by means of small tingles, or with a stapling gun (Fig. 58).

Lacing Method. To secure the leather by lacing, holes are made round the margin by the use of a leather punch. The leather is drawn over the margins of the cast and secured by a criss-cross lacing with twine, a loop being tied over the anterior portion of the cast to secure the forward end of the leather. A transverse portion of the lacing is used as a point of anchorage from which fanwise lacing secures the portion of the leather brought over the heel. Care should be taken to see that the leather is smooth and free from pleats round the margin of the heel.

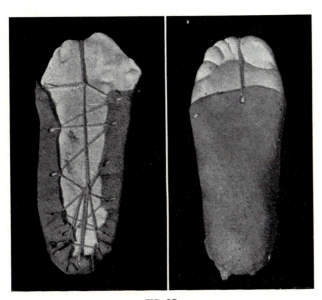

FIG. 57

The method of lacing the basic leather in position.

Tingle Method. Another satisfactory method of securing the leather is to use small lasting tingles (small sharp tacks). The leather can be drawn over the edges of the cast with a pair of crocodile pincers (lasting pincers). These have a square hammer head under the base of one of the jaws which is used for driving in the tingles. The tingles should only be driven partly home, so that the heads stand proud. This is requisite as it may be necessary to remove tingles from time to time during the stretching-over process to improve the fit of the leather; it also helps when the appliance is finally removed from the cast.

Stapling Method. This method has been introduced as being the quickest and most convenient method of securing the leather.

I

The stapling gun is operated by a lever which acts like the trigger of a gun, releasing the staple which is punched by the spring-loaded mechanism into the leather and pinning it to the cast. When it is desired to remove the appliance from the cast, this can be done by levering the staples out with a small screwdriver or other suitable instrument (Figs 45 and 58).

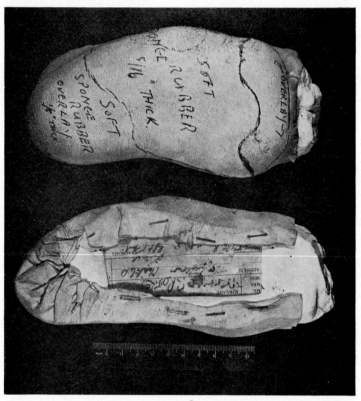

FIG. 58

Soaked basil leather stretched onto cast of foot and stapled with staple gun. Note. Identification slip set in plaster before setting and making up instructions written and drawn on leather.

Laminating

When the leather has been thoroughly dried, the laminations should be applied. These are of an open-weave fabric. A suitable material is scrim which is a very coarse open-weave canvas made from jute string. Cotton bandage is a very satisfactory material to use for laminating but being very thin, a considerable number of laminations will be necessary if this material alone is used (Fig. 59).

Appliances combining both scrim and cotton bandage are now made as the result of experiments which showed that the strength and non-fracture qualities of the cotton bandage, and the ability of the scrim to hold a considerable quantity of the cement, enabled an appliance to be produced that was reasonably thin and not prone to fracture.

I will now proceed to describe the application of the laminations in all three types.

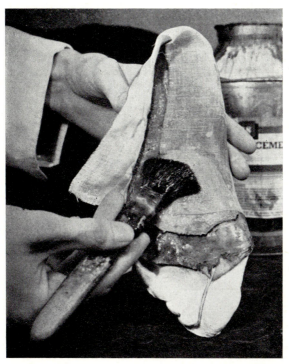

FIG. 59
Applying a cotton bandage lamination.

First Type. In this type, seven laminations of scrim are used with the addition of two small pieces of the material. These strengthen the area of the first metatarsal-cuniform articulation, as this is the area of greatest stress in the long arch weakness (pronation).

In applying the laminations, first commence by applying a coat of Pochin's cellulose cement evenly over the leather. The lamination of scrim is laid onto the leather and gently pressed into the cement. The index and second fingers are now used to rub down the fabric, bedding it well down onto the leather, ensuring that the cement has fully engulfed it and filling the spaces in the open meshwork of the fabric. This procedure is assisted if the fingers are dipped in the solvent for this cement, as they will glide smoothly over the fabric without sticking to and lifting the cement.

This technique is repeated until five laminations have been applied, when the two strengthening pieces are put on after which the remaining two laminations are applied.

The reinforcing pieces are applied across the first metatarsal cuniform articulation as this is the point of greatest stress in the corrective insole in particular. It can be made still stronger at this point without thickening the whole appliance, by inserting a strip of spring steel about $\frac{1}{2}$ inch wide and $2\frac{1}{2}$ inches long with a hole at each end. The reason for the holes is that the cement and fabric are pressed into them and thus secure the spring which is, of course, in place of the reinforcing strips of fabric.

When all the laminations are firmly in place, the edges can be lifted and trimmed down to approximately the shape and size intended for the finished appliance. When this is done, the laminations are pressed back in position and finally rubbed down.

The appliance should be put on one side in a dry place for at least twenty-four hours, after which it can be removed from the cast (Fig. 60).

The next stage is to do any further rough trimming with strong scissors or small shears and complete the final shaping on a scouring wheel.

Second Type. The second technique is the cotton bandage technique, and here the most important point to remember is that each layer of the material must become thoroughly impregnated with the cement. Eighteen to twenty laminations of open-weave cotton bandage will be required for this type when used in a corrective insole for mobile pronation, but a strong wafer-thin appliance is possible as a double flanged cradle type insole for pes cavus, using only twelve laminations, the processing technique being the same as in the scrim appliances. An alternative method of applying these laminations is to start with a longitudinal lamination and then apply transverse laminations, each overlapping half their width (Fig. 59).

Appliances made in this way are probably the strongest of all and only slightly thicker than the previous type.

Third Type. This is the type in which the scrim is sandwiched between layers of cotton bandage.

First apply three layers of cotton bandage and follow this by applying two layers of scrim and complete with three more layers of cotton bandage. Even four layers of scrim will not make the appliance unreasonably thick, but the practitioner may vary the laminating as a matter of experiment, increasing or decreasing the number of laminations in either fabric.

It should be remembered that the object of using scrim is that the coarse meshwork of the fabric provides a means of retaining the maximum amount of the cement, several layers of the material

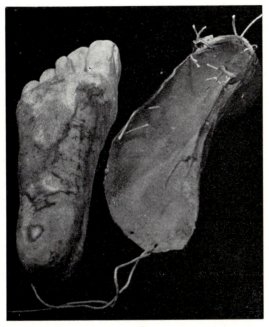

FIG. 60

The string lacing is cut and the appliance removed
from the cast.

forming a meshwork in depth in which the maximum quantity of the cement will be retained even when the rubbing-down process has been finally completed.

The cotton bandage is used because it is strong and thin and is less liable to fracture under stress.

In the processing of any of the types described, it is important to give a final pressing down about one hour after applying the laminations.

The cement is a transparent syrupy fluid which, during its fluid state, tends to float the layers of material away from each other. If left to dry without the final pressing down, the appliances would be thicker and weaker with a degree of sponginess. The object in leaving the appliances for one hour after laminating is to give the cement time to set partially so that when pressed down by rubbing firmly with the ball of the thumb, the laminations become firmly fixed together and remain that way.

It will be noted that when carrying out this final rubbing down, beads of water from condensation will be present on the surface which will act as a lubricant during the process.

These three types each have their own merits. The first type made entirely of scrim is quick and easy to make and quite strong. The area of the long arch can be further strengthened if desired by further pieces of scrim, as can the outer flange. This may be necessary when it is desired to extend the outer flange to act as a strong buttress to receive and hold severe lateral pressure, as in the case of an appliance for talipes varus.

The second type, made entirely of cotton bandage, is probably the strongest and lightest appliance devised and is particularly useful where the minimum of bulk is desired. It is highly suitable for use in smart footwear either as a flangeless insole, or with a low medial flange.

The sandwich type is probably the most useful type, as it has the minimum of bulk consistent with the use of flanges.

In the making of laminated insoles the cellulose cement is apt to harden on the fingers and to be difficult to remove later. Rubber gloves are unsuitable as a protection as the solvent attacks the rubber but the appearance on the market of thin, cheap, disposable plastic gloves solves the problem of hand protection during laminating. If these gloves are found to be rather hot in use they can be ventilated by punching holes in the back.

The laminated corrective insole has the advantage of being light in weight, resilient and positive in its corrective action upon the mobile foot. It is, however, very important that the cast upon which the appliance is made is accurate, incorporating the heel spread of the weightbearing heel with the fully reformed arch achieved by the corrective manipulation when casting. There is no doubt that putty casting is the most suitable technique for the production of a cast to be used in the making of corrective insoles for mobile pronation.

Trial Fitting

Before finishing the corrective insole a trial fitting in the patient's footwear is necessary. The reason for this is that footwear conforms to the dictates of fashion to varying degrees; also the appliance, when first made, will have considerable surplus material which must be removed by scouring (Fig. 61). It must be remembered that the basic feature that the appliance requires for correction is that it should in the first place have been made on a cast of the corrected foot, and that it should have a cupped heel and a strong lateral heel flange to take the thrust that will be exerted upon it as the heel tries to fall into eversion on weightbearing.

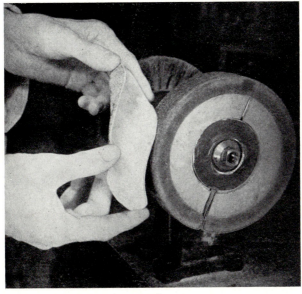

FIG. 61

Shaping the appliance on the scouring wheel. (Alternative technique.)

The conventional medial flange should not be exaggerated, that is to say bigger, than it need be, but at the same time it should not be reduced to a point where it will fall under the medial arch with the foot on weightbearing, overriding it and causing it to dig into it.

The lateral flange will have to take severe stress only at its base and therefore its upper margin can be thin and flexible so as not to impinge uncomfortably on the side of the heel or beneath the malleolus.

The insole of the shoe is usually shaped to swerve in behind the position of the great toe joint, making the waist portion somewhat slim.

If the anterior portion of the medial flange and the forepart of the support do not follow this inswerve, it will be found when the appliance is fitted into the shoe that this portion will override onto the upper, preventing it seating properly on the floor of the shoe. The posterior margin of the medial flange likewise should be curved well in to keep the appliance as narrow as possible across the anterior aspect of the heel, otherwise the upper will be pressed out and make the shoe fit badly. The anterior margin of the appliance should extend to immediately behind the head of the first metatarsal, curving forward behind the head of the second metatarsal then back behind the remaining metatarsals to finish behind the fifth.

Some practitioners prefer the appliance to be made as a full sock device to distinguish it from the standard commercial arch supports. This is a matter for the individual to decide. If made as a full sock it cannot slip forward when the shoe is being placed on the foot, but if the shorter appliance is carefully fitted to the shoe and has a rubber gripping piece under the forepart, there will be no difficulty with slipping.

Fixing the external covering leathers is the last part of the job. The upper or inside leather is adhered first and its edges are turned over the edge of the appliance all round (Fig. 62). These edges are pressed down and any wrinkles cut off. The turned-over edges are now roughened and thinned either by hand or on the scouring wheel to provide a key for the outer or under leather which is then applied. The edges of this are brought up to the edge of the appliance and cut off flush. These covering leathers are applied with rubber solution and it is desirable to select two contrasting colours. The lighter coloured leather goes inside against the foot. A black leather outside and a white one inside probably make the best combination.

Cushioned Surfaced Insoles

Laminated insoles can be cushioned either by applying rubberzote or foam rubber sheeting to the superior surface of the appliance. When this is done the insole is covered with fine kid or basil leather in a suitable colour (cream, beige or white), the under surface being covered with a material of a more serviceable colour.

If $\frac{1}{8}$ inch foam is used to cushion the surface, the leather cover will seal it in and form a pneumatic cushioning effect which is very soft and kindly to the foot. The rubberzote is a little firmer in texture but it is very springy.

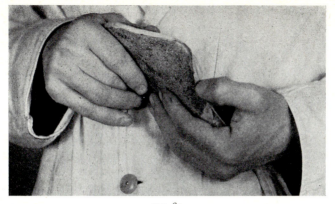

FIG. 62

The top leather being secured in position.

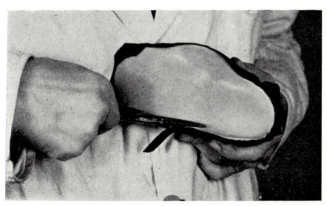

FIG. 63

Trimming the bottom leather.

Cushioned Forepart

It is frequently desirable to provide support and cushioning round painful pressure points on the ball of the foot whilst keeping the appliance as thin as possible. In this event, the forepart can be cushioned in a simple form by applying the cushioning material to the anterior portion of the appliance, only scouring away its back edge with the scouring wheel.

Before making the insole requiring forepart cushioning for metatarsal symptoms, it is as well to remove some of the plaster close round the area to be supported so that the appliance will exert a greater supporting pressure in these areas. The overlying rubber will cushion this.

Two-texture Rubber Technique

A technique has now been evolved to provide the softest possible surface to be presented to the foot, whilst underlying this is a firmer material giving positive support. This is achieved by making the appliance in the following manner.

A piece of fine soft textured leather should be secured over the cast which has been previously prepared by scraping out the plaster round the pressure areas and the metatarsal area generally. The skin is dampened before it is stretched on, and when in place on the cast it is well rubbed down round the pressure areas to ensure that it fits perfectly to the cast. When the leather is dry a layer of $\frac{1}{8}$ inch foam rubber is applied with rubber solution, extending from the base of the toes to the base of the metatarsals. The next step is to apply a piece of rubberzote of appropriate thickness to give adequate support, this material being shaped with cut-outs to allow it to fit close round the prominences. These are bevelled so that they will mould round the pressure areas without ridges at their margins.

When the rubber is in place, the edges are bevelled away on the scouring wheel, a gradual bevel being made at the posterior edge of the padding. When this is completed, it is sealed in with a piece of thin leather, the upper surface being roughened with sandpaper so that the cement used in laminating can key into it.

The laminating is now carried out using the Pochin's cement and one of the laminating fabrics according to which of the three types is required.

The appliance, when finally shaped on the scouring wheel, can be finished with a covering of suitable soft leather, i.e. fine Persian suede, London finish (cream), beige or white kid. A two-tone finish is again most pleasing, using a dark more serviceable colour for the under-side of the appliance. The covering leathers are secured by the use of rubber solution. It is a good plan when scouring the appliance to thin the base of the heel seat as much as possible so that the heel of the foot will not be raised too much in the heel seat of the shoe, causing it to slip when walking.

Trial Fitting

It is important not to put the finishing leathers on the appliance before a trial fitting has been carried out, as it is important that the insole should fit snugly in the shoe if it is to give satisfaction.

Where arthritic changes have occurred making very prominent painful pressure areas, the padding technique may be modified as follows:

Apply the first layer of $\frac{1}{8}$ inch foam rubber up to the base of the toes. Now cut out the rubberzote support padding to extend over the pressure areas to about $\frac{1}{4}$ inch beyond. Now mark the pressure areas on the rubberzote and cut apertures in it corresponding to the pressure points. The next step is to secure the rubberzote in place with the pressure areas seated in the apertures. To complete the padding cut out foam rubber inserts to fit the apertures, and of sufficient thickness to fill them completely and secure them in the apertures with rubber solution.

With this combination you have the thin insulating carpet of $\frac{1}{8}$ inch foam rubber extending to the base of the toes to take any over-ride, the rubberzote of adequate thickness to provide the necessary supporting padding, and finally the foam inserts to ensure that on extreme weightbearing, soft cushioning protection is ensured for the painful pressure areas.

Forefoot padding may be required in combination with a corrective insole from time to time, more particularly in a case of pes cavus.

THE CORRECTIVE LAMINATED INSOLE FOR MOBILE PRONATED FOOT

The appliance for the correction of mobile pronated foot may be made either all in scrim or as the sandwich type of insole. It is so designed that on weightbearing it induces the foot to assume the corrected position with the heel inverted and the forefoot everted thus reforming the natural arch of the foot. This is done by making the appliance with a cupped heel seat and a substantial lateral flange. This appliance will also have the normal type of medial flange.

As the device is made on a cast of the corrected foot it should seat firmly on the three-point bearing, namely the base of the heel and points just behind the plantar aspects of the first and fifth metatarsals.

As the foot is placed in the shoe the heel will be guided into the inverted position by the lateral heel flange. When a weightbearing stance is assumed, the forefoot will bear down upon the forepart of the appliance everting the forefoot and depressing the head of the first metatarsal.

The ideal shoe and appliance combination for the mobile pronated foot is one in which the lateral flange of the appliance is extended but gradually diminishes up to the base of the fifth metatarsal. This will ensure that the foot is retained in its correct position on the floor of the shoe as the extended flange will prevent a side-slip of the foot away from the medial arch. It will, however, be necessary to choose a shoe with a good broad waist, a strong shank and a firm heel counter.

This combination provides little difficulty in men's footwear and children's shoes, but it is more difficult in the case of women on account of fashion.

For an adult a broad-waisted walking shoe with a heel not exceed-ing $1\frac{1}{4}$ inches is most suitable, but in the case of adolescents and young children the 'nature-form last' children's shoe is ideally suited. The principle of treating children by the use of appliances has in the past not been regarded with favour. Whilst many of the milder cases of long arch weakness in children correct themselves without treatment, many cases of severe pronation not only fail to correct in this way but by neglect result in other complications—round shoulders, pigeon chest, defective gait, etc. This new form of plastic appliance is extremely light, and has the right degree of resilience. It does not interfere with normal foot function, but by holding the foot in correct position assists in re-education in walking, and by establishing stability, a normal gait is assured.

In the course of experiment and development of these appliances they have been employed effectively in young children of $2\frac{1}{2}$ years of age and even younger. Orthopædic surgeons who are now familiar with these appliances are unhesitatingly prescribing them for children.

Adults under treatment with this system of correction may, if desired, be fitted with a specially modified pair of insoles for wear on social occasions when more fashionable shoes are indispensable. It is strongly urged that such modified insoles should always be worn when the fully flanged appliance is not in use. This should, however, be resorted to as infrequently as possible, the fully flanged insoles being worn continuously for all general purposes.

The Modified Type of Insole

The insole can be modified to fit the more fashionable narrow-waisted shoe by reducing the inner flange in height and length. The flange, however, should extend to just beyond the navicular. From this point the medial side of the insole can be shaped to a curve toward the lateral side, the anterior platform of the appliance being just wide enough to provide support beneath the first metatarsal. The lateral flange can be dispensed with, leaving only the outer buttress. This, however, should be as strong and firm as in the normal insole. It will not be necessary to reduce the general strength of the insole, and care should be taken not to weaken the anterior platform or medial flange. On no account should the appliance be modified when treating mobile pronated foot in adolescents or children.

THE HEEL PITCH MACHINE

In making these appliances for shoes with heels of more than 1 inch in height, the author advises that the casts should be made by the slipper casting technique, and the foot placed on the heel pitch machine invented by the author and described in Chapter 2 (Fig. 12).

This machine is particularly useful when making light rest appliances to wear in ladies' shoes. The practitioner cannot always have what he desires when undertaking these cases and may have to compromise in the matter of footwear. It is surprising what can be done with the use of the heel pitch machine and some degree of co-operation on the part of the patient in this matter.

Summary. It is as well to consider the use of a power-driven scouring wheel for the trimming and shaping of the appliances. The writer has used a $\frac{1}{4}$-h.p. motor to drive a small shaft fitted with sandpaper wheel and carborundum wheel quite satisfactorily.

The cement may be applied with a 1-inch soft bristle brush. The brush will set quite hard in a very short time after use, but if placed in a jar with enough solvent to cover the bristles it will soften out in a comparatively short time.

The appliance should be allowed to dry out as long as possible before removing from the cast for finishing, and on no account should the chiropodist be tempted to rush the work, as quick drying or finishing before being properly set will lead to distortion. The finished appliance, when quite firmly set, should be fitted to the patient as soon as convenient, as it is not advisable to have them lying about for long periods since it is possible that a further shrinkage of the cotton reinforcement will exaggerate the curve of the long arch. This tendency is a good thing, however, when the insole is in wear, as it strengthens the resistance to flattening under weight-bearing.

The practitioner should take into account the weight of the patient and the severity of the pronation when deciding upon the strength of the reinforcement required. It is particularly important in relation to the anterior portion of the medial flange and the base of the lateral buttress. These appliances have been fitted to obese patients, weighing in the region of 17 stones, with complete success when care has been taken in the design and making of the appliance. Adequate reinforcement can be applied without unduly increasing either bulk or weight.

9

Palliative Surgical Insoles

PALLIATIVE INSOLES

PALLIATIVE insoles were devised to provide light insoles moulded to casts of the feet that would provide a degree of support and weight distribution and would also cushion and protect pressure areas on the plantar surface of the foot. These insoles were mainly devised to wear in ordinary stock shoes and even moderate types of fashion footwear.

These insoles are fashioned as a light, surgical sock made using either the cotton bandage technique or the sandwich type. The object is to make them very light and thin so that they will, while giving a measure of support diffused over the whole plantar surface of the foot, mould into them the required extra cushioned support and protection of the painful pressure areas. These appliances have proved particularly helpful in chronic metatarsal pain involving plantar corns and callosities under the heads of the metatarsals (Fig. 66, *top right*).

They are often designed as a moulded flangeless sock, thin but reasonably strong with a cushioned forepart. The cushioning is, as has already been described, light $\frac{1}{8}$ inch foam extending from the base of the metatarsals to the base of the toes. Rubberzote, also $\frac{1}{8}$ inch thick, is shaped to support the area behind the painful pressure areas and extend over them with bevelled apertures in which the pressure points can sit, with the firmer rubber supporting the painful areas. When the rubber has been prepared it should be placed in position and a pencil mark made round it. It is removed and the leather within the pencilled area coated with rubber solution. The rubber pad is coated also (Fig. 64). When the rubber solution is dry, the padding is carefully pressed into position, after which it may be finally shaped on the scouring wheel (Fig. 65).

The extent of padding in this type of appliance is limited by the restricted accommodation available in the shoe, but the firm sock helps to support the forefoot and thus, by taking some of the load, reduces the amount of padding required.

The laminated sock only extends to the base of the toes, the foam padding extending forward as a soft flexible flap to the base of the toes to take any override.

This type of appliance can be varied in strength according to the degree of accommodation so that, in a comfortable type of walking shoe, it can be designed to give considerable support perfectly diffused over the whole plantar area of the foot and particularly under the forefoot. In fashion shoes for occasional wear, the appliance can be wafer-thin but still capable of relieving the painful pressure area under the ball of the foot.

For wear in smart shoes, this type of appliance can be covered with fine champagne-coloured or white kid on the upper surface and a Persian suede on the under-surface.

Semi-flexible Cushion Insole

This type of insole is designed as a pneumatic rest insole for geriatric cases in which degenerative changes in the tissues have resulted in keratotic masses over pressure areas resulting in a painful and crippling condition (Fig. 66, *bottom*).

For this appliance, putty casting is particularly useful. It is, however, desirable to have impressions with the indents of the pressure areas enlarged. This is achieved by the use of a sheet of $\frac{1}{8}$ inch rubberzote, used as described in the putty casting section, being placed on the surface of the putty so that a corresponding larger imprint is obtained. The resulting cast from this impression is now covered with a very soft leather which is dampened and stretched over the cast, being pressed closely to the contours of the excrescences. When the leather is dry, a sheet of latex foam is solutioned on to it after which metatarsal padding with apertures as previously described is applied along with valgus padding.

The foam overlay can be from $\frac{1}{8}$ inch to $\frac{3}{16}$ inch according to the amount of cushioning desired. When the padding has been appro-priately bevelled by scouring on the sandpaper wheel (Fig. 65), the whole is sealed in by a layer of thin skiver secured with rubber solution. The next stage in the process is to apply three layers of cotton bandage laminations with cellulose cement.

When dry the appliance is removed from the cast and finally shaped to fit in the selected footwear. This should be roomy and made of soft leather such as kid. Felt boots are often very useful for these patients and accommodate the appliance well.

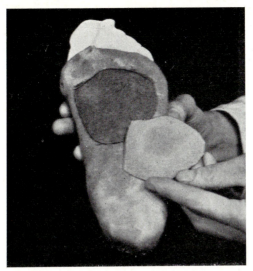

FIG. 64

Area marked out and solution applied, the metatarsal pad about to be secured in position.

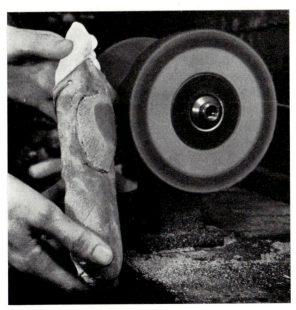

FIG. 65

Shaping a metatarsal pad on an emery wheel.

K

When finally shaped to fit, the appliance is finished with a top cover of fine soft leather and an under-leather of suede.

When sealed in by the covering leathers, this appliance is very light and softly cushioned. As well as being very flexible it gives just the right measure of support.

Being moulded to a cast of the foot, the appliance will diffuse all the pressure away from the painful areas. This type of rest insole is designed expressly for the geriatric patient whose footwear is suitably roomy and which will accommodate the appliances adequately.

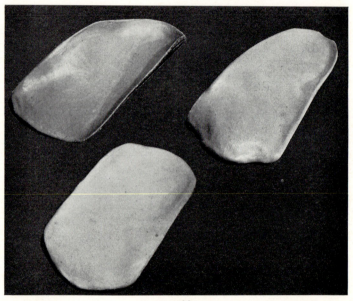

FIG. 66

Examples of surgical insoles. (*Top left*) corrective insole; (*top right*) metatarsal rest appliance; and (*below*) a cushioned surface rest insole for arthritic flat foot.

Made in this way these appliances are firm and strong whilst, at the same time, they provide moulded cushioning soft enough to relieve painful unyielding prominences.

Care must be taken not to make any insole surface too soft. If this should be done the patient sinks deeply into the sponge cushioning which yields under weightbearing. One of two things then happens. Either the prominences press through the cushioning on to the sole of the shoe and are painful, or movement of the cushioning under the foot in walking makes the patient unstable. Both these faults are to be avoided. This basic factor underlies the whole principle of this technique.

By using the putty casting method, a faithful reproduction of the plantar aspect of the corrected foot can be achieved. The materials used in this manufacture ensure an exact relationship between insole and foot. In this way a reforming and stabilising foundation can be perfected, providing rest and eventual readjustment of affected ligaments. Progressive remedial exercises, Faradism and other forms of physiotherapy are often a necessary adjunct to the treatment, improving muscle tonus and assisting in re-establishing structural and postural stability and normal function.

In the rest appliances, the establishment of a firm stabilising foundation and resilient support, with complete diffusion of weight-bearing eliminating pressure points, are vital factors in treatment. This is achieved by the combination of the sponge rubber pads with cotton laminations. Again, the basic principle of the appliance is that the individual characteristics of the foot are interpreted faithfully.

It must be stressed that the method of impression taking described in an earlier chapter is an integral part of the making of the final appliance. No adaptation made in the process of making-up will correct errors of impression taking as these will be transferred to the cast on which the appliance is being made.

The technique of processing is straightforward but the basic needs of the patient, whether they be comfort and protection or relief of strain and correction, must be constantly borne in mind so that the appliance can be designed and made to provide for these needs.

Both the short- and long-term results are good. Comfort and relief of strain can be provided from the beginning. The effects of protection are seen later in the diminution of callus and corn formation and in the improved skin texture in atrophic cases. Correction is maintained to the extent and in the manner explained in Chapter 8.

Surgical Sponge Insoles

There are occasions when soft resilient surgical insoles are desired to give a degree of resilient cushioning to the long arch and to the anterior metatarsal area. It is realised that appliances of this nature have been manufactured for many years, but as in the case of other types of surgical insoles, complete accuracy in fitting is not possible unless these appliances are made on individual casts. There have been occasions when this type of appliance has been found appropriate to the case and, as a result, efforts have been made to evolve a technique that will produce a really satisfactory appliance on these lines.

For this type of appliance a plantar cast admirably meets the case. A soft, resilient leather is first carefully stretched over the cast. Chamois leather is very appropriate for this purpose. It should be stretched tightly over the cast and should be drawn and stretched at every point so that each prominence and depression is accurately embraced. As an alternative to this leather a soft basil split may be used. In stretching this leather great care will have to be taken, as it tears quite easily if roughly handled. It will be found advantageous to damp the leather on the underside, as after dampening it stretches more easily. The leather should, however, be only lightly damped and not made thoroughly wet, and when stretched over the cast it can be laced or stapled on. The next stage in processing the appliance is to apply a thin coating of rubber solution all over the leather.

When this is dry firm sponge rubber or rubberzote is fitted to the area where special support is to be provided, that is, a valgus pad under the instep or padding round painful pressure areas in the metatarsal region. When this padding has been shaped and fixed into position, it may be carefully trimmed with scissors or scoured with an emery wheel as in other types of appliances. Another coat of rubber solution is now applied. A sheet of thin surgical sponge is shaped to cover the whole plantar area of the cast. The side which is to contact the cast is lightly scoured to ensure the adhesive obtains a firm hold, after which this side is given a coat of rubber solution. When the two surfaces are tacky, this thin sheet of rubber is fixed in position, after which the margin is carefully skived to avoid a thick edge. Again, this may be done with a high-speed emery wheel, if available. A piece of fine soft basil split is trimmed to shape, solutioned on the underside, laid in position and smoothed down over the plantar surface of the appliance.

When completed, the appliance may be removed from the cast and the surplus trimmed off. The result will be a soft and resilient appliance which will fit accurately to the foot, giving a soft, cushioning support. The appliance is principally palliative in effect, but as in all such appliances once relief and comfort have been established the patient will use the feet with greater confidence and tend to resume a more normal gait. This is bound to have its effect upon circulation, muscle tonus and the re-establishment of muscular balance, making for improved function.

This type of appliance is often improved by making it in the form of a full sock. To do this the leather stretched on the cast should be allowed to extend well beyond the toes, although it should only be secured to the same extent as the half-sock appliance. If the lining sock of the patient's shoe can be removed it may be used to ascertain the total length of the appliance and as a guide for shaping the sole part. In processing the appliance the medial arch should be fitted with the rubber valgus pad, after which a full sock of thin surgical sponge should be secured from heel to ball, leaving the sole portion extending forward insecured. Any final scouring and shaping of the half-sock portion of the appliance should be completed, after which the final leather bottom cover is secured in place again only up to the half-sock. To complete the appliance it is now removed from the cast and the unsecured portions of top and bottom leathers secured to the rubber sole part, which is finally shaped with scissors to the size and shape of the insole of the shoe.

Sponge Rubber Supports

Flexible appliances of this type are frequently referred to as non-rigid supports, but we feel that this term is somewhat misleading. It is assumed that metal appliances and others that present a firm unyielding surface to the foot are designated 'rigid', but many of these appliances possess a degree of springiness which assists the normal action of the leg muscles and can in consequence hardly be classed as rigid. It is therefore advisable to refer to appliances made from soft spongy materials by a descriptive title other than that of non-rigid.

One type of sponge rubber insole has been described which was moulded onto leather stretched over a cast of the foot. This type of appliance, by the very exact nature of its construction, is the most efficient form of support moulded from surgical sponge rubber. Whilst, however, the sponge rubber appliances are soft and comfortable to the foot, their effectiveness is dependent on soundly constructed shoes that are well balanced and have stronger rigid shanks.

A much simpler type, however, can be made, which if carefully designed and constructed will prove very beneficial in many cases where mechanical correction or support has to be of a limited character. The sponge appliance can be made in a variety of ways. They may take the form of simple inserts solutioned to the insole of the shoe and covered with soft basil leather or kid, or may be constructed in the form of a full-length surgical sock or half-sock, with the pads secured in the appropriate places.

INSERTS

Sponge rubber inserts may take the form of metatarsal pads, valgus pads, a combination of both, or heel pads. It will be realised that pads of this type depend upon accurate fitting for their effectiveness, and the chiropodist must apply himself with painstaking diligence to designing the shape, thickness and position of these pads.

Valgus Pad. Where the treatment of pronated foot is contemplated, a combination of valgus pad and medial heel wedge is desirable. A drawing of the outline of the foot should be taken with the patient seated. The drawing should be marked to indicate the position and length of the long arch. The length of the foot from the back of the heel to the head of the first metatarsal should be measured with calipers.

The sponge rubber should be of moderately firm consistency. Latex foam will be found too soft for this purpose; $\frac{1}{4}$ inch rubberzote is quite suitable. The pad is built up of two parts. The sole piece is shaped to go under the arch of the foot from just behind the meta-tarsal heads to the back of the heel and passes well up on the medial side. A further D-shaped piece is superimposed on this with the round curve of the D passing up under the medial side of the arch. The pad is now bevelled all round. A long bevel is made on the lateral border of the heel piece to give the heel wedge. The insole of the shoe is now cleaned with petroleum, ether, or some other suitable spirit-cleaner to remove dust and grease, after which it is roughened with sandpaper.

The insert is now secured in position with rubber solution, and the operation is completed by covering it with an insole of thin soft basil leather.

This form of insert may be made by first completing the valgus pad and heel wedge separately. They are then fitted separately in the shoe.

Another form of valgus pad incorporates a plantar metatarsal pad. Again, it is a more simple method to shape the metatarsal pad and valgus pad separately, and then fit them in the shoe in their proper relationship.

The object of the valgus pad is to lessen the strain on the inverting muscles and to reduce the strain on the supporting ligaments. Strain on the plantar fascia is also reduced by this form of valgus pad.

A modification of the pad is made by cutting a circular piece of sponge rubber bevelled away to the margins, the equivalent to placing D shapes with straight edges together. A deep V-shaped cleft is cut down the centre of the upper surface of the circular pad. The cleft is treated with rubber solution and its sides brought together, forming the pad into a right angle. This form of pad not only supports the navicular but exerts a lateral thrust against it. The heel wedge is designed to tilt the heel with the object of bringing the calcaneum from eversion to an upright position.

When fitting inserts incorporating a valgus pad it is important to ensure that it extends over the whole area of the dome of the long arch. The heel wedge should be sufficiently broad to extend to the middle of the heel seat of the shoe. It is not easy to calculate the exact thickness required for the valgus pad, as the curve of the shoe waist has to be taken into account, and some degree of experiment will no doubt be necessary even when the accommodating qualities of the soft tissues are allowed for.

Pes Cavus Insert. A useful and simple form of insert for pes cavus to assist in achieving a uniform distribution of pressure is to fit a pad of sponge rubber in the waist of the shoe. The rubber pad should be bevelled away at the anterior and posterior ends, and should be of sufficient thickness to fill in the space between the long arch at its outer border and the floor of the shoe. The pad should extend the full length of the arch, and the calipers should be brought into use to ensure that it is properly placed. The lining sock should be removed from the shoe before inserting the pad, and should be refitted over the pad.

Metatarsal Pads. In designing plantar pads for metatarsal defects, it is advisable not only to pad directly behind the area to be relieved and supported but to provide both anterior and lateral insulation. The pad fitted in position to the pressure point deflects pressure, whilst the thin insulating padding cushions the wider area. The most satisfactory method of constructing a pad of this type is to shape and fit the deflecting pad and superimpose the broader insulating cover over it. Care must be taken when fitting to press down and secure the cover anterior to the deflecting pad so that the necessary hollow is provided. The insulating cover should extend to the base of the toes.

Whilst single and double wing pads are frequently quite effective in this type of insert, a more complicated pad requiring a very precise positioning is not on the whole very satisfactory in this type of fitment. They require the foot to be securely anchored in relation to them, and the play in the shoe will usually allow the foot to become displaced in relation to the pad, and result in much discomfort to the patient.

Heel Pads. A sponge rubber insert, however, is very satisfactory for the relief of calcaneal spur. A more satisfactory method than the conventional aperture in the pad at the site of the spur is to cut a deep hollow in the pad on the underside. This is treated with rubber solution as well as the whole under-surface of the pad. When being fixed it is pressed down firmly in position at the point of what is now an inverted hollow or dome. This will make a permanent depression with smoothly rounded sides, but with a thin soft layer of rubber as a final insulation against pressure on the tender area on weight-bearing. When this pad has been secured in position a thin soft cover of basil or kid will complete the job. A pad of this nature but without the depression will, on occasions, prove adequate in the treatment of achillo-bursitis, by lifting the affected area clear of the back of the shoe.

Shaping and Bevelling. If sponge rubber pads are to be comfortable and effective, it is necessary that their shaping and bevelling should be accurately and neatly carried out. Trimming with scissors is a method which requires much skill and painstaking application if the pads are to be cleanly shaped and smoothly bevelled. It is quite a good plan to fit pads that have been bevelled with scissors, with the flat side uppermost, as when fixed in position the soft flexible material shapes itself in reverse and in this way a clear smooth surface is presented to the foot. It has been found that the most satisfactory method of shaping sponge rubber pads is by the use of a power-driven emery wheel revolving at a fairly high speed. The type of wheel used is one as used on a shoemaker's finishing machine. The wheel is in two halves, hinged together. It is made of wood and has a layer of compressed felt round it. The emery paper is fitted round the wheel by engaging the ends of the strip on metal spikes fitted near the rim of the two halves of the wheel. The two parts are closed, which tightens the emery strip upon it. A locking device is screwed home and the whole is firmly secured. The one used was modified to go on a small stand fitted with 'V' pulleys, and the results have proved most successful. Pads shaped by this method have a really well-finished appearance, and make this inexpensive and simple piece of machinery well worth while, especially as it is a valuable piece of equipment for the processing of many other forms of appliances.

It is most important to cover all sponge rubber inserts with a soft thin leather. If this is not done they will cling to the foot, either preventing its fitting properly into the shoe or the pad will be dislodged in the attempt to insert the foot in the shoe. Whilst latex foam rubber is very soft, fine in texture, and most comfortable, it is not suitable for use in inserts, as its extreme softness allows it to be depressed too completely on weightbearing, and as a consequence the thickness required for adequate cushioning is too great for use in the form of inserts, and this material does not lend itself to shaping by use of the emery wheel.

Sock Appliances. Socks, or insoles as they are alternatively called, are the basis of a form of simple appliance which has been in common use for a great number of years. The form of padding used in appliances of this type is in the main similar to that used as inserts which have already been described. The sock type merely consists of building the padding onto a leather sock which can then be inserted into any shoe. This, of course, obviates the fitting of several sets of inserts into the various shoes of the patient.

The sock should be sufficiently flexible to press down and mould itself to the contours of the shoe insole, whilst being sufficiently stiff to avoid curling up at the back of the heel. A very satisfactory method of making a surgical sock is to use two pieces of leather, a firm piece—a piece of fleshing will do—and a soft kid or basil top leather. The sock should be an exact replica of the insole of the shoe. This is necessary if undue play is not to occur in wear, causing a malpositioning of the padding.

A simple way of taking a pattern of the shoe insole is to cut out a piece of paper of sufficient length and width to fill the shoe insole with some to spare. Place this paper in position, taking care to press it well into place, then get a pair of closed scissors or other suitable instrument and run the point round the margin of the insole, pressing sufficiently firmly to crease and mark the paper, but taking care not to tear it. When this is accomplished the paper should be carefully removed from the shoe and trimmed along the crease, outlining the insole. This pattern can be used in cutting out the leathers for the insole. If the shoes are new and possess a leather lining sock, this can sometimes be removed and used as a guide for shaping the sock. It should be noted that a generous margin should be allowed when cutting out the top leather, as it has to be folded over the outline and thickness of the padding.

When leather and padding are shaped, they are assembled by first securing the padding in position on the bottom leather, after which the top leather is carefully moulded over the padding and secured firmly to both padding and bottom leather. If all portions have been secured by a good rubber solution or latex milk rubber, the sock should stand up to reasonably hard wear. If desired, a row of stitching can be carried round the edge of the sock to give further strength and finish.

Care in positioning the padding is most important, and the calipers are a most useful instrument for measuring from the back of the shoe heel (inside) to the points of pressure or anterior margin of valgus pad or P.M.P.

In some chronic cases it will be found advantageous to fit deflection padding in position and then cover the whole sock with thin surgical sponge, finishing with a covering leather. This simple form of appliance is inexpensive and frequently proves quite adequate.

As in the case of inserts, the form of padding used is based upon previous experience with the patient with felt or surgical sponge in the normal course of treatment.

Cork Wedging. A very simple and inexpensive form of sock appliance that can be used as a replaceable sock or be permanently fixed in the shoe is made by using fleshing for the sock and cork for the wedges (Figs 67 and 68). Fleshing is loose offal removed from the underside of bend leather, compressed and impregnated with a stiffening substance. This form of leather is very cheap, but nevertheless makes a firm, clean material for the sock. A sock of this type makes a very useful appliance for contra-lateral wedging (inside heel and outside sole wedge). The cork wedges can be secured to the under-side of the sock by a good rubber solution. If desired, the finished appliance can be secured in the shoe in the same way. The use of cork for these wedges results in a very light appliance and has proved quite satisfactory. In the appliance referred to, the sole wedge should extend from the centre of the toe of the shoe and cover the whole half of the sole. The wedge should graduate away to a paper edge in the middle of the sole, so that any suggestion of a ridge is avoided. This method of wedging, whilst being simple and inexpensive, is not quite as effective as wedges inserted between the middle sole and outer sole. The discrepancy is that the internal wedge causes angulation at the midline of the sole and heel. The insole method, however, is a useful alternative where difficulties are encountered in getting the work carried out or the problem of expense arises. The insole may be fitted with medial cork heel wedge only for mild pronation, and this type of appliance is useful used as a lateral heel wedge when a buttress is required in the case of a weak ankle. Leather wedges may be substituted for cork if desired or if found more practicable for any reason. If a softer or more pliable surface than a fleshing leather is required cortex sheet makes a satisfactory alternative.

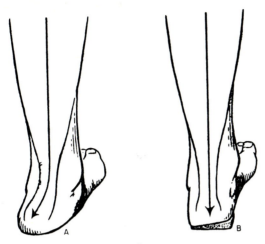

FIG. 67

A. Showing eversion of heel and inswerve of tendo-
Achillis when foot pronated. B. Showing corrective
effect of wedge. Heel is inverted.

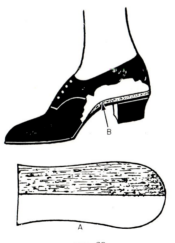

FIG. 68

A. Underside of cork wedge showing cork
extending mid-way across leather heel sock.
B. Cork wedge in shoe (medial side).

I O

Surgical Inlays and Contact Therapy (American)

SURGICAL INLAYS

The American Dynamic Inlay Technique

THE word inlay is being used here to distinguish the type of appliance made within the shoe by means of a plastic impression compound which ultimately becomes part of the final appliance, from those which are moulded on a plaster cast. The technique has largely been developed in America and although the principle on which it is based differs somewhat from the British one, it is advisable that it should be understood along with the methods employed to carry it out, as it has much merit.

The dynamic inlay is an insole appliance which is made by putting a plastic compound in the shoe itself, often in a polythene envelope. The shoe is placed on the foot and worn for a considerable period of time, at least three hours, after which the appliance is taken out of the shoe and put to one side to set fully. After this it is trimmed and finished on the scouring wheel and covered with the appropriate soft leather. If the compound is to be moulded and cured in the shoe, a polythene sock is placed over it before the foot is placed in the shoe. At the end of the specified time, when the foot is removed, the polythene sock is taken out and replaced by a leather one.

The principle here is one of displacement of the volume of plastic compound which is placed in the shoe to a level of about ¼ inch. As the foot presses down into it, the compound displaced under the pressure areas flows into the concavities of the foot, thus providing stability and support; the depression made by the prominences or excrescences are there to receive them so that when the compound is set, the foot is retained by the surrounding medium, relieving them from pressure.

It has been found advisable to enlarge the concavities so that they are a little bigger than the actual prominences to eliminate friction. This is done with a nail drill using a suitable burr after the compound has hardened.

There is one type of shoe made in America which has a separate insole with a lip round the edge in which the compound is placed. The sock is then replaced in the shoe and a process similar to that already described is carried out.

These shoes are made in the appropriate size and fitting so that the patient will have adequate room.

The author has tried the appliances described, not the shoe, and found the pressure under the arch rather severe so the appliance had to be discarded. The conclusion from this was that too great a volume of compound was used and it is not quite clear how one arrives at the correct amount required for each individual case except through experience. There is, however, considerable success with these inlays in chronic cases requiring rest appliances, and one feels that this technique may be profitably explored by British practitioners.

The plastic compounds used in America are of formulæ secret to their inventors but latex milk rubber, ground cork, leather dust and wood flour are all used in the making of moulded inlays. Experiments were therefore carried out to test the consistency and texture of plastic compounds suitable for this work. The author made up formulae varying the quantities of the appropriate ingredients. Leather dust was found to be a most suitable ingredient inasmuch as it was light and soft and readily absorbed the latex milk. Wood flour, according to the proportion used, tended to make the finished product less resilient but gave it a firmer texture. Ground cork made it very light and reasonably soft. The purpose of cork would appear to be twofold: to lighten the weight of the finished appliance and, not being absorbent, reduce the quantity of latex milk in a given quantity of the plastic compound. It should, however, be noted that not being absorbent, the latex does not adhere to it very firmly but rather imprisons the granules. Therefore, if used in excessive quantities, the finished product does not wear so well since the granules will tend to separate out and fall away, certainly on the surface areas of the appliance.

A formula at present being used by the author is to add the latex milk to ten ounces of leather dust, four ounces of wood flour and two ounces of ground cork. This can be mixed in a stainless steel or plastic bowl until a consistency of a stiff paste is reached that can be easily trowelled but will not tend to creep or run.

Corrective Insoles

As in the case of the laminated appliance a cast of the corrected foot is used, and if there are no excrescences the use of a mat in the impression-taking is not required (p. 130).

A soft leather is dampened and stretched upon the cast, being secured by stapling or other suitable method. To prevent the superior surface of the skin from becoming stained by a seepage through of the latex milk which contains ammonia, the leather is given a coat of rubber solution before the compound is applied. In fact, the author prefers to apply one coat, let it dry, and then apply a second coat. When applying the compound the object is to fill in the contours of the arch, square up the heel margin carrying the compound up the side of the heel on the lateral side of the heel and the medial arch so as to form flanges similar to those in the laminated appliance.

It is important that the edges be squared off forming a clean, sharp buttress so that the appliance will be stabilised on the floor of the shoe when fitted. Reasonably generous quantities should be applied as when set the appliance will be ground down with a scouring wheel to the appropriate thickness to provide a smooth, even finish.

On the plantar surface the compound should be scoured to wafer-thinness under the base of the heel, along the pressure area along the lateral side of the foot and across the anterior metatarsal area—in fact the actual weightbearing surfaces of the natural foot. The scouring should not be done until the compound is thoroughly cured by a natural drying on the cast from which it should be removed before the scouring is undertaken.

Before commencing the scouring the appliance should be trimmed down to its final shape providing a cupped heel, a lateral heel flange and a medial arch. The appliance may extend to the heads of the metatarsals or it can be made as a full sock appliance if desired, in which case the portion anterior to the metatarsals should be very thin so as to take up as little room in the shoe as possible.

If the process is correctly carried out, the surface of the leather should be unblemished and the appliance is ready for trial fitting. A suitable shoe with a strong waist should be used, that is one with a good shank. Flexible-waisted shoes for this purpose, unless they are heel-less shoes, are not advisable.

A good finish to the appliance may be obtained in a variety of ways. The discoloured appearance of the composition may be coloured either by the application of a coat of cellulose paint or soft Persian suede leather. Another method is to cover the appliance with a thin sheeting of a rubber and cork composition which is very popular as a base for metatarsal socks and valgus socks. This can be solutioned round the sides of the appliance and on the bottom, after which it is buffed down to the thinnest possible dimensions on the fine scouring wheel until a fine, light-brown mat finish results.

This looks very well and also prevents slipping along the insole of the shoe.

Another method is to use very thin white rubber composition sheeting. This is applied and used in a similar fashion. Again it is scoured down to the thinnest possible dimensions. This gives a beautiful milk-white finish providing a non-slip surface, both appliances having a nice, soft leather surface next to the foot making an appliance with a very presentable appearance.

CONTACT THERAPY

Another form is the contact mould which is another name for what we have referred to as a dynamic inlay. This appliance, developed by Samuel Rosoff Pod. D., was described in the *Journal of Podiatry*, October 1953, and has since been used successfully by the originator and many of his colleagues.

He described the contact mould as an appliance formed by direct contact with the foot under dynamic conditions which, of course, is the same in principle as appliances we have already described as dynamic inlays. This represents a foot in the shoe rather than one in free space and is claimed to be a composite of all foot attitudes rather than a static device representative of only one attitude of the foot.

Rosoff claims that with so many radical tissue changes between the foot in free space and the foot encased in shoes, it is virtually impossible to get an accurate transference into the mould made over a free cast. He, very wisely, insists that as a preliminary to the use of the contact mould the patient should be relieved of all pain symptoms, muscular spasm, oedema, etc. as far as possible.

He takes care to ensure that the patient's shoes to be used for his moulds have the necessary accommodation. Otherwise, he advocates that new shoes should be fitted.

A felt platform is cut to the size of the sock lining to avoid bulk at the perimeter. He prepares a thin latex mixture with equal parts of latex and water in an enamel pan to a depth of 1 inch. He then prepares a mixture of rubber butter by mixing two ounces of latex with sufficient wood flour to make a thick butter and adds a pinch of plaster of paris to accelerate setting. The felt is immersed in the thin latex which is allowed to saturate it thoroughly. The excess is then squeezed out. It is smoothed out and the rubber butter is spatulated on. The amount and its position will vary according to the indications of the individual case, taking into account the depth of the shoe and the deflection of the foot under weightbearing.

These, and any other relative factors, will vary the amount and positioning of the rubber butter.

Two pieces of surgical stockinette are now required, two and a half times the width of the felt and 2 inches longer. The surgical stockinette should be lightly dusted with plaster of paris.

The felt is now placed with the side coated with rubber butter downwards onto the stockinette. The stockinette is now fabricated into an envelope, care being taken not to distort the original shape of the felt. The device should present a smooth, wrinkle-free surface. The inside of the shoe is wiped round with liquid paraffin to prevent adhesion of the mould to the side of the shoe when drying takes place. As an alternative, a wax paper lining may be used. The mould is carefully slipped into the shoe and a wax paper cover applied with a posterior tail-piece that is held by the patient when the shoe is slipped on the foot to prevent its being pushed forward in the shoe.

Before slipping the foot into the shoe, it is lubricated with an emolient cream, no stockings being worn by the patient. The patient is now instructed to plantar flex the toes several times and to walk round the room for five minutes. When the shoes are removed it will be noted that a crested mould has been formed.

The patient is instructed to return in several days. The moulds set in about forty-eight hours. During this period the patient must not remove them from the shoes. When the moulds are properly set they can be removed and worn in other shoes provided they are of a similar type and form to the ones in which they were originally made. Any excess of latex in the shoes may be removed with a stiff brush.

Rosoff points out that as the moulds have been worn more or less constantly during the drying process, shrinkage is minimised. These moulds make a light, long-wearing appliance. It is claimed that they dynamically and hydraulically compensate for the imbalance. Being contained in the stockinette envelope, it is claimed that a measure of hydraulic compensation takes place wherein the fluids under pressure or body weight are forced into areas of least resistance.

Dynamic inlays and contact moulds as described by Rosoff are extensively used by our American colleagues. There is much truth in the criticism levelled by Rosoff of appliances made to casts, but there has been considerable advance in appliance therapy in Britain and modifications in casting technique have been introduced which have eliminated a great deal of the cause for this criticism.

The author has recently produced appliances resulting in the marrying of British and American techniques which are proving exceptionally successful. Convenience of processing and perfection of finish leaves little to be desired in these new appliances, referred to as surgical inlays. They are being extensively used by many British practitioners who have trained in his department at Hope Hospital, Salford, and the numbers fitted in the Foot Orthopædic Clinic run into several thousands. These are discussed in the next chapter.

THE MOLO PLANTAR MOULD

An alternative method of making a dynamic inlay employs Molo, a soft compressible rubber sheet which, when cut to the size of the insole and inserted in the shoe, takes an impression of the foot during wear.

A sheet of this material, about $\frac{1}{16}$ inch thick, is sufficient unless there are marked protuberances and heavy lesions on the sole of the foot.

This Molo insole is covered on its upper surface with leather and placed in the shoe. The patient is then instructed to wear the shoes as much as possible for about a week. On return a good dynamic impression of the sole of the foot is found. A plantar metatarsal or arch pad can now be added in the same material if necessary and the patient told to wear the shoes for another week. Further additions or corrections can be made as necessary either by adding more layers of Molo or by deepening indentations with a rotary file. These enlarged indentations can be plugged with foam rubber if a sensitive plantar lesion demands softer cushioning.

This method, although not available in Britain at the time of writing, has the advantages of being less messy and easier to apply than the use of paste impression compounds which tend to get extruded into the rest of the shoe.

Molo is a compressible material comprising certain gels, leather and cork bound with a special formula latex. It moulds itself under weightbearing to the contours both of the foot and the insole of the shoe. The indentations so made do not spring back and the impression once firmly made, is permanent. The appliance can then be covered with thin leather which can be adhered with rubber solution.

L

II

Moulded Inlay Techniques (British)

BRITISH PRINCIPLES

The American dynamic inlay or contact appliance is formed by direct contact with the foot, and is based on principles already outlined under the headings of Surgical Inlays and Contact Therapy (pp. 142 and 145).

The moulded inlay developed by the author is based upon a cast of the patient's foot. The cast can, however, be produced by a technique that will, in the opinion of the author, provide adequately for the tissue changes considered in the dynamic inlay technique.

In the case of the corrective insole for pronated foot or for the treatment of foot-strain symptoms, the putty casting technique has proved quite successful, as the patient's foot is manipulated into correction in the process of taking the negative impression, and a semi-weightbearing stance is adopted.

When making stabilising or rest inlays for chronic cases in which painful excrescences or prominent pressure areas are involved, two methods of casting are available to the practitioner. One is to use the putty casting technique, making a deep impression and using a rubberzote mat $\frac{1}{8}$ inch thick over the putty (p. 130). To prevent it from sticking, dust the surface of the putty slab liberally with french chalk. The impression produced will be oversize and less sharp than a direct impression into the putty.

This oversize impression is necessary as the painful areas should sit easily into the depressions in the finished appliance. The type of foot we have under consideration has little mobility and tissue changes will be limited as movement will be very restricted.

The footwear of this patient will be designed to accommodate the appliances rather than the appliances modified to fit the footwear.

If, however, the appliances are for a less severe case in which reasonably fashionable footwear has to be considered, casting by the slipper casting technique is advisable, coupled with the use of the heel pitch machine, as the finished inlay must be moulded to suit the heel height and waist curve of the shoes to be worn. The slipper cast will restrict the tissues on weightbearing to a similar degree experienced in footwear, but care must be taken to straighten out the toes when making the slipper cast, so that they are not restricted when weightbearing.

As soon as the slipper is completed, the foot should be placed without delay on the heel pitch machine which has been pre-set to the required heel height. A mat of $\frac{1}{4}$ inch sponge rubber is placed on the machine so that the foot sinks into it allowing the excrescences, etc., to stand out in the finished cast.

The positive cast is now made from the negative as it is upon this that the appliance is moulded.

The Composition

The composition from which these inlays are made consists of latex milk, leather dust, wood flour and ground cork. The practitioner may experiment in the varying quantities of the different ingredients used to make up the composition. The proportion at present used by the author is as follows: to make one pound in weight of the dry compound use ten ounces of leather dust, four ounces of wood flour and two ounces of ground cork.

The leather dust is the basis as it is very absorbent, fusing freely with the latex. The wood flour makes for a more solid, harder composition and the ground cork merely provides bulk with extreme lightness. As the ground cork is not absorbent, the cork granules are merely imprisoned in the latex and if used in an excessive quantity they will tend to separate from the general mass. Ground cork should only be used as a means of keeping the appliance light in weight, and the quantity used in the formula given has proved satisfactory.

When the leather dust, wood flour and cork have been weighed out they should be well mixed together so that a good, even balance is obtained in the mixed compound. A stainless steel or plastic bowl is now filled to a depth of about 1 inch with latex milk and the ingredients, which have been well mixed together, are added, being whipped into the latex with a flexible steel spatula, until a sufficient quantity has been added to produce a soft dough which, whilst spreading freely with the spatula, will not tend to run.

The compound should only be mixed when required although the ingredients, other than the latex milk, can be mixed in quantity and used as required.

Making the Corrective Inlay

These, as in the case of the laminated insoles, are made upon casts of the corrected foot. A soft sheepskin leather is wetted and stretched over the cast and secured by stapling or other suitable method. When dry the leather is given two coats of rubber solution. This is to prevent the latex soaking through and staining the upper surface of the leather. The next stage in the process is to apply the moist compound by spreading it on with a spatula. To help in the final spreading, the compound should be gently patted with the flat blade of the spatula. This causes the latex milk to come to the surface when the blade can be lightly stroked over the surface.

The concavity of the medial arch should be filled in and a flange built up with the compound by spreading it thinly up the medial side of the leather. The compound should be trowelled over the plantar surface to a depth that will fill in the waist curve. The average covering of compound will be about $\frac{1}{8}$ inch. A flange should be built up on the lateral side of the heel. The outer margin should be squared off with the base of the heel to form a buttress. The whole of the heel margin should be treated in the same way, as should the outer margin of the whole appliance. The compound should be spread over the whole plantar surface to extend beyond the metatarsal heads.

The appliance is now placed in a warm, dry place to cure, which takes about three days, after which it can be removed from the cast and trimmed to shape with scissors.

The next stage in processing the appliance is to scour the rough under-surface removing all excess material, finishing with a clean sharp edge at the heel margin and shaping in the medial arch to form a waist curve that will sit on the floor of the shoe without riding on the upper. The appliance should be scoured very thin under the heel and along the lateral border and ball of the foot. The anterior margin of the inlay follows the posterior margin of the metatarsal heads.

When shaping the medial arch flange, care should be taken to get a good inswerve, both anteriorly and posteriorly to prevent its pressing out and riding on the side of the shoe. When finished, this appliance should sit firmly on the floor of the shoe, have a deeply cupped heel seat and a lateral heel flange about $\frac{3}{4}$ inch deep at its highest point with the bottom margin forming a slight buttress. The medial arch should be ground to an incurve, the base following the line of the insole along the curve of the waist, the appliance standing firm and stable on the insole.

The inlay type of corrective appliance requires a shoe with a rigid waist, as, unlike the laminated insole, it will sag down with the flexible waisted shoe on weightbearing.

This appliance has been found, if carefully shaped and fitted in a rigid waisted shoe, to be one of the most effective means of treating foot-strain symptoms, and can be strongly advocated for the treatment of patients whose feet are subject to excessive static strain.

The corrective inlay is particularly suitable for the treatment of mobile pronation in children, as the appliance is light, kindly in application, takes up little room in the shoe, and can be used for very young children.

For clinical use, where cost must be kept down as much as possible, no further finish is required as the somewhat muddy, drab colour of the compound is not visible when the appliance is in wear, and the fresh-looking London finish sheepskin top leather is quite pleasing. The compound can, however, have mixed with it a little ground colour in dark brown which would give it a more pleasing finish.

The appliance can, however, be made with a first-class finish by covering the top leather with a suitable fine skin and the under-surface and sides with a Persian suede, in fact a variety of finishes can be contrived by a combination of contrasting top and bottom leathers. If this superior finish is to be carried out, a very thin split leather will suffice for the top leather.

A further development of this technique evolved by workers at Hope Hospital, Salford has been to stretch well-soaked blocking shoulder or belly leather onto the cast instead of the soft basil leather. This needs to be held in place on the cast with $\frac{3}{4}$ inch tacks and to be well rubbed down or lightly hammered into the contours of the arch. When dry the latex milk paste compound is applied as previously described and subsequently scoured on the grinding wheel. The appliance is then removed from the cast, shaped, finished and fitted.

This method produces a much stronger appliance capable of applying correction to the foot and resisting deformation under stress in the shoe. The stability it engenders in the foot is often equivalent to that obtained by means of the laminated surgical insole to which it makes an acceptable alternative.

Cradle Inlay

Another successful inlay appliance is the cradle or double-flanged inlay. This is used for the cavus deformity. The appliance is made in the same way as the corrective insole except that a very deep putty impression will be required for the cast.

This appliance is made with a cupped heel and deep flanges both medial and lateral. Again, care must be taken to see that the lower margins of the flanges sit on the insole and do not override it.

The only problem with this inlay is one which besets all double-flange appliances, namely the width of the waist. An appliance with two flanges needs a broader waisted shoe to accommodate it than is required for the single-flanged appliance. It is, therefore, important that both the shaping of the appliance to fit the floor of the shoe without overriding onto the uppers and the width fitting of the shoe should be given careful attention.

The Metatarsal Inlay

This type of inlay provides plenty of scope for variation to cope with each particular problem, from painful callosities over the second metatarso-phalangeal joint, to a painful first metatarsal callosity or sesamoiditis.

In this type of appliance, metatarsal support can be exerted at a particular point by exaggerating the depression behind a particular pressure area by scraping out some of the plaster on the cast. This will mean that the greater depression caused by this operation will be filled with compound providing increased support at this point.

When the metatarsal area is very painful, it will be advisable to provide cushioning and also to take into account the tendency to overriding, which can be done by making a metatarsal insole with a cushioned forepart and an extension to the base of the toes. $\frac{1}{8}$ inch latex foam is a suitable material.

Cushioned Forepart with Extension

In making this appliance, the areas round the painful points should be scraped out to increase the support at these points. The skin selected to cover the cast should be soft and supple, so that when wetted it can be stretched on and moulded into every depression.

When the leather has dried, it should be coated with two layers of rubber solution, and a layer of $\frac{1}{8}$ inch foam rubber applied extending over the whole metatarsal area to the base of the toes. A pad is now cut in rubberzote, which is a firmer textured sponge rubber, and shaped to fit close round the pressure areas. The margins should be bevelled so that they can be fitted very close, even impinging up the sides of the prominences. This pad is solutioned in place, after which the padding is scoured to obtain the correct amount of bevelling leaving the maximum padding to provide the necessary support and cushioning. By applying the first layer of

$\frac{1}{8}$ inch foam rubber, a final base of soft cushioning at the points of greatest pressure and a forward carpet to provide insulation against the overriding is provided.

Excessive padding should be avoided and the whole plantar area stabilised by applying the subsequent layer of latex paste compound in the arch area and over the whole plantar surface, thus achieving diffusion of pressure as far as possible. If the padding is sealed in with a piece of thin leather secured with rubber solution before the compound is applied, the forefoot padding will have a pneumatic quality which will make the appliance more comfortable.

This appliance can be finished as the previous ones by covering in suitably thin soft leather. A very excellent material to finish the plantar surface of the appliance is the thin rubberised cork sheeting (Cortex). This is about $\frac{1}{16}$ inch thick. It can be applied on the bottom of the appliance and then scoured down to a wafer thinness; this provides a firm, light brown mat finish which is non-slip. This is a very useful material for the plantar surface of all the inlay type of appliances.

An alternative to this is $\frac{1}{16}$ inch white rubber sheeting which can be used in the same way. This, like the cork sheeting, can be scoured down to paper thinness and gives a very clean non-slip finish.

In applying covering leather the upper leather should be applied first (Fig. 62) and it is advisable to apply the plantar cover before the side and flange covers as in bending a plantar covering up to the sides the appliance will be distorted. The side portions should, therefore, be applied separately and last and the edges brought neatly together. After this it will be found that on buffing down, the joint will be almost invisible, and the appliance will have a slightly firmer quality which will not easily distort, whilst standing up to wear and tear even better, and yet retaining that flexible quality which makes this appliance so kind to the feet.

The Rest Inlay for the Chronic Case

This appliance requires the cast to be taken to suit the type of patient and the footwear. If the patient insists on reasonably fashionable footwear, the practitioner's scope will be limited but if the excrescences are very prominent and painful a cushioned surface will be necessary, and the indentations in the appliance to receive the painful prominences will have to be adequate to receive them.

The positive cast will be produced by first taking a slipper cast using the heel pitch machine, or alternatively using shaped cork blocks to support the heel and the instep to the required heel height.

It is better to use a heel pitch machine as a rubber mat of adequate thickness will have to be placed upon it.

When applying the plaster bandage, care should be taken to apply it loosely. Massage the creamy plaster through the mesh of the bandage and mould the bandage round the prominences. The toes should be held in the stretched out position when applying the plaster bandage to ensure proper function. The foot is placed on the rubber sheet on the heel pitch machine before the plaster has had time to set, and a weightbearing position should be taken up, only moderate pressure being applied.

The positive cast is covered with a soft, pliable leather, care being taken to ensure that it is moulded round the prominences and into concavities. The leather is next coated with rubber solution.

A sheet of $\frac{1}{8}$ inch latex foam is now applied with solution to cover the whole surface of the cast, after which a piece of rubberzote is cut to shape, the apertures corresponding to the excrescences or painful prominences. The rubberzote should be sufficiently thick to come well up the sides of the prominences with the apertures appropriately bevelled. When secured in position it should be graduated away, blending with the underlying foam rubber. The whole can now be enclosed by applying some thin skiver; small pieces can be used. They can be joined together when applied and this will use up scrap pieces.

The compound is now applied and moulded up level with the summit of the excrescences and prominences. When the curing period has been completed, the appliance can be removed from the cast, trimmed to shape and buffed down to the required thickness. The appliance can be finished with the cork or rubber sheeting.

Shoes should be made with the measurement taken round foot and appliance. This combination has proved most successful in long-standing chronic cases where other methods have given little relief.

It should be noted that these appliances are further assisted when equal care is taken in designing the footwear.

12

Blocked Leather Surgical Insoles

THIS is the oldest form of foot support, and was usually made by the bespoke boot-maker for a customer who complained of foot pain, particularly if a marked flattening of the foot occurred on weightbearing.

The blocked leather insole was also frequently prescribed by doctors for patients exhibiting symptoms of long arch weakness. The appliance takes the form of a full-length insole with a flange on the inside. The material used is light, vegetable-tanned sole leather which has been soaked in water overnight. The leather is laid along the sole of the last from heel to toe and secured by two rivets. The leather is then drawn tightly over the sides of the last with lasting pincers, and secured with tingles (small sharp tacks). The leather is beaten lightly with a hammer and gradually moulded to the last. The tingles are released and the leather drawn tightly on to the last from time to time until firmly shaped. The beating of the leather compresses the fibres making its texture more compact, and as a consequence firmer and stiffer.

The moulding of the leather is assisted by rubbing with what is called a lick stick. This is a piece of hard wood or bone, and is usually used for burnishing. When the sock has been shaped onto the last by stretching, beating and rubbing with the stick, it is left on the last to become thoroughly dry. When removed from the last the insole is found to be firmly blocked to shape, after which it is finally trimmed and skived round the edge on the underside with a leather knife (Fig. 69).

This form of insole can be further improved if a leather wedge is fitted on the medial side of the heel portion. The wedge should extend to the middle of the heel seat and should be about $\frac{3}{8}$ inch thick, graduating to nothing. Care should be taken to avoid forming a ridge down the centre of the heel where the wedge terminates.

Blocked leather insoles are also made for pes cavus, the object, as in all rest appliances, being to diffuse pressure.

The appliance is often made more effective by making depressions in the insole to receive the painful callosities beneath the metatarsal heads. Insoles of this nature are designed with both an inside and an outside flange, and are usually cemented firmly in the shoe.

Whilst this method of processing surgical insoles is perhaps the oldest, it is still used by surgical and bespoke boot-makers, and is much more effective than many of the commercial appliances which have not the advantage of being made so near to the shape of the patient's foot.

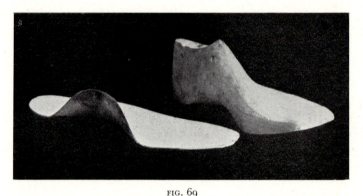

FIG. 69

Showing blocked leather insole and the last upon which it was made.

Metal Reinforcement of Surgical Insoles

It has for many years been the practice to reinforce blocked leather surgical insoles by the means of metal, the materials most commonly used being steel pressings, aluminium or German silver. Recently German silver and similar metals have not been used, and reinforcement is confined in the main to the use of steel or duraluminium.

In the use of reinforcement of surgical insoles, one has to consider the object of the appliance. If it is designed to provide a flexible support that will allow some degree of flexibility, the only satisfactory material is spring steel. In the case of rest appliances of chronic cases where the object is to give firm support and stability and where the absence of flexibility is not detrimental, the most suitable material is duraluminium because it is both strong and light. Malleable metal may be used quite effectively, the only difficulty being the added weight.

Reinforcement of this nature may be used either in the old type of blocked leather full or half-insole support, or in a similar insole strengthened by the use of cellulose cement. In certain cases requiring strong rest appliances the author has embodied a duraluminium supporting strip into the cork and cement compound in the appliances made by this process.

Flexible Spring Steel Reinforcement

Spring steel is not a particularly easy commodity to obtain, but an engineer's shop can usually supply it. It should be remembered that it is only a reinforcement and not the whole support, and should in consequence be light and well tempered. One method of obtaining a supply of suitable material is to purchase an old clock spring or spring from a gramophone motor. Springs varying from $\frac{1}{2}$ inch to $\frac{3}{4}$ inch width made from about 22 gauge metal would be suitable.

The method employed by the author to fix this form of reinforcing strip is as follows: cut a length of spring steel about $\frac{1}{2}$ inch to $\frac{5}{8}$ inch wide of sufficient length to bridge the medial arch. To ascertain the required length, the strip of steel is bent against the medial arch of the plaster cast. It should be held so that it passes beneath the first metatarsal under the navicular to the anterior aspect of the tuberosity of the calcaneum. When the correct length is procured, it is held in the flame of a Bunsen burner or blow-lamp until cherry red, the metal being grasped at each end by pliers. When sufficiently heated, the metal is placed against the cast in the previous position and bent to the required curve and held in this position until it has cooled off and turned black. The metal is again heated until cherry red and then plunged into oil. The spring will now have regained its temper. should it be overtempered and brittle the temper can be adjusted by reheating. The heat required this time should be only sufficient to burn off the oil: again return it to the oil to cool and this will adjust the temper of the metal, but it will have retained its curve. The next stage is to drill two holes about $\frac{1}{4}$ inch from each end, also corresponding holes in the leather, after which the spring is secured in position by two aluminium or copper rivets. This form of reinforcement will be found most useful and will add to the life of the appliance considerably. The important point is to remember that the spring should be light and very flexible (Fig. 70).

In the case of rest appliances requiring strengthening, a strip of duraluminium, about 22 gauge, will be very suitable for quite a substantial support. The metal is curved to fit the cast by gently bending with pliers and beating with a rawhide hammer until it fits the cast perfectly. The metal strip is then drilled and secured in the same way as already described.

It is interesting to note that the late Thomas Holland, well-known arch support manufacturer, claimed that his father invented the first arch support, which consisted of a block leather surgical sock with a metal spring reinforcement. This appliance was first made and patented well over one hundred years ago.

Blocked leather insoles can also be made of saddler's leathers, cowhide bag leather or what is termed as strap leather, and blocking (moulding) shoulder or belly leather of 1.5–2 mm thickness.

The leather is wetted and stretched on the cast with a pair of crocodile lasting pincers. These have long, narrow, curved, serrated jaws. At the base of the lower jaw is a square piece of metal which is used for tapping the leather down or driving in the small sharp tingles which are used to hold the leather at the point to which it has been stretched. The careful stretching and moulding of the leather onto the cast is assisted by light hammering and rubbing down with a lick stick or bone.

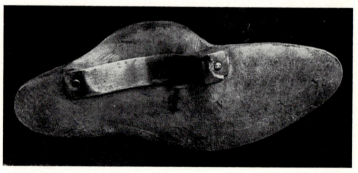

FIG. 70

Blocked leather surgical insole reinforced with spring steel.

The tingles are not driven completely home during the stretching process as they have to be removed from time to time during the stretching-on process. When exerting gentle lever action on the leather whilst stretching over the cast, the small hammer head on the lasting pincers can be used as a fulcrum.

When stretching leather onto a last it can be hammered and worked on vigorously. However, when stretching leather on a plaster cast one must proceed more gently. The moulding is achieved by gently stretching with the pincers and pressing with the ball of the thumb. Tapping with the hammer head is liable to fracture the cast but an ash hammer handle may be used safely.

Another method of stretching strap or blocking shoulder leather onto a cast in the making of a block leather appliance is to stretch on first with the lasting pincers and secure at a limited number of points with tingles, after which a strip of rubber is used to press it firmly to the contours of the cast and compress it. One end of the rubber is anchored and the rubber strip is bound round the leather under considerable tension, each turn of the rubber strip half over-lapping the previous one until the whole area is covered. The end of the rubber strip is then secured after which the appliance is laid by to dry out.

When dry the appliance is cut to its final shape, replaced on the cast and suitably reinforced. This reinforcement may take the form of laminations of cork sheeting, cork and rubber compound as used in the moulded inlays, or fibreglass.

A further form is the use of cellulose gum and several layers of cotton bandage. This combination makes a very firm and light reinforcement. To my mind it is an improvement on fibreglass as it is not quite so rigid.

An apparatus can be devised similar to the shoe-maker's stake which stands upright on the working bench to hold the last. The leathers can then be blocked on positive casts made from slipper casts in which dowels have been inserted before setting to allow the cast to be dropped into place with the plantar surface uppermost, leaving the operator to work freely with both hands.

There are a variety of ways in which equipment of this kind can be devised for the easy attachment of the cast during the leathering and reinforcing process. Incidentally, a piece of bicycle inner-tube is very suitable for the rubber binding strip.

Reinforcement

The earlier types of block leather insoles made by the surgical boot-makers were considered self-supporting. Sole leathers were used and, being moulded on wooden lasts, they could be beaten and rubbed down until the leather was sufficiently compressed to ensure their retaining their shape even under the pressure of the foot. As we have already described, in certain cases where they were likely to be submitted to extreme pressure, they were reinforced with spring steel.

However, those made from bag leather are not so strong and although they are reasonably firm and retain the shape to which they are blocked, they require some reinforcement. A variety of materials have been utilised for this purpose and it depends upon the degree of resilience desired as to what material is used.

One method of reinforcing the arch is to build it up with lamina-tions of sheet cork. This makes a fairly rigid support but one that is very light. Building up the laminations of cork sheeting is more convenient than shaping a piece of block cork. By building in the laminations they follow the natural curve of the arch, and when the arch curve has been reinforced with sufficient laminations it can be finished off with a scouring wheel. In the case of block cork it means that one has to keep shaping the block to the exact contour of the arch before fitting, a difficult process.

The laminations are secured by the use of rubber solution or cellulose cement. If the laminations are not going to fill in the whole of the arch, to allow a degree of resilience they should be secured with cellulose cement as this adds strength whilst retaining the resilience.

Another method is to use a compound of latex and leather dust. Again, the appliance is considerably lightened if ground cork is introduced into the composition.

Another and most successful method of reinforcing this type of insole is by the use of cellulose cement and cotton bandage. This has many advantages inasmuch as it can provide very strong reinforcement whilst retaining a considerable measure of resilience. Also, the amount of strengthening and degree of resilience required can be very accurately controlled by the number of laminations applied. Another factor in favour of this method is that even when sufficient laminations have been applied to give very considerable strength to the appliance, little bulk has been added. The reinforcement will have set hard within twenty-four hours and it can be scoured and feathered away neatly at the edges eliminating any ridges. In most cases three or four laminations are adequate. It is important to note that when supporting the insole with any form of lamination or composition, it should be firmly secured to the cast during the operation and until the materials have completely dried out, otherwise shrinkage will cause distortion.

Another material which has now been introduced is fibreglass. This is probably one of the strongest reinforcing materials and is very effective if a rigid appliance is required.

After lengthy experiments and clinical experience of these various methods of reinforcement, it seems that cotton bandage and cellulose cement laminations are the simplest and most effective.

In certain cases of metatarsalgia where severe, painful excrescences are not in evidence, the block leather insole can be designed to provide a metatarsal support in addition to valgus support. If the cast is hollowed out immediately behind the metatarsal heads extending backwards and shallowing off midway up the metatarsals, it provides for the necessary doming when the leather is blocked on-to it. This can be filled in with rubberzote or with composition paste (latex and leather dust, etc.). If the depression is to be filled with rubberzote it can be made more resilient if desired by making the leather much thinner in the dome area by scouring before apply-ing the rubber.

The practitioner can vary the shape, degree of elevation and resilience of his metatarsal support to meet any special requirement.

Blocked leather insoles have a neat and trim appearance, are hard-wearing and are very efficient in the less complicated cases.

The Double Surface

A factor that is worthy of careful consideration is the importance of stabilising the appliance in the shoe, as this must be achieved if the foot itself is to be stabilised.

Whilst the superior surface of the appliance fits faithfully to the cast upon which it has been moulded, the inferior surface may present several protuberances and depressions which would seriously interfere with the proper stabilising of the appliance in the shoe by causing it to tilt and rock. This problem can be overcome by present-ing a uniform flat surface to the floor of the shoe where pressure is received. This can be achieved either by filling in the depressions until a level surface is reached, by using a compound of cellulose cement and cork fillings, or by using leather skivings secured with rubber solution. A perfectly uniform surface can finally be obtained when the filling is set, by scouring with an emery wheel or sandpaper block. It is also a good plan to square up the curved margin of the heel by the same method.

13

The Whitman Brace

THIS corrective foot appliance was devised by Dr Royal F. Whitman and originally described in the *Medical Record* of 31st August 1907. The device is made of malleable metal, i.e. duraluminium and malleable steel or stainless steel, and consists of a medial flange and lateral flange piece which acts as a clip. Unlike the standard arch support with a forward edge curving transversely across the heads of the metatarsals, the Whitman brace cuts obliquely across the foot from the base of the fifth metatarsal to immediately posterior to the head of the first metatarsal. The absence of a heel seat is also a feature in which the appliance differs from other surgical insoles.

The Whitman brace is unique in its corrective principles. The patient is directed to place his weight on the lateral side of his foot which rests upon the appliance. The resultant lateral thrust causes the appliance to tilt and raises the medial flange, pressing it against the inner side of the foot, and causing the foot to be drawn away from this point of pressure. In this way the foot is caused to be drawn up into its normal contours, reforming the long arch. The patient does not evert the foot, as to attempt to do so would cause considerable discomfort. Any relaxation of the foot will again induce pressure from the medial flange, so that in effect the patient can only walk in comfort when the foot is held in the corrected position. In this way the brace induces a corrective stance, and when walking the patient is in effect carrying out a compulsory corrective exercise. The appliance has, therefore, a positive action in the physiological correction of pronation.

The author suggests that instead of correcting a cast of the foot by rasping plaster away beneath the arch as directed by Dr Whitman, a corrected cast be taken as for the corrective appliance technique.

In shaping the appliance the medial flange should curve up to a point just beyond the tuberosity of the navicular. In the foot with a naturally low arch curve, however, it is advisable to bring the flange a little higher. When making the brace the practitioner should start by taking a cast of the corrected foot. This may be done either by the putty casting method or by slipper casting. As the medial flange in this device extends well up the inner side of the foot, care should be taken in the case of putty casting to obtain a deep impression. Whichever method of casting is used, correction should be obtained by inverting the heel, everting the forefoot and depressing the head of the first metatarsal. When a satisfactory cast has been obtained, an outline of the shape of the appliance should be placed upon it, after which a paper pattern is cut to act as a template,

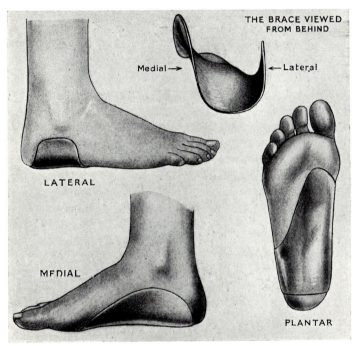

FIG. 71

A Whitman brace.

which is used in marking out the shape of the appliance on the metal. When the metal has been cut out in rough shape, it should be curved by the use of a mallet and lead block to fit the contour of the long arch of the cast. This is achieved by a slow beating process. When the metal has been beaten to the correct curve of the long arch, attention is paid to the lateral clip and medial flange. A vice will assist in bending the lateral clip to some extent, but the medial flange can only be successfully moulded by the metal beating process.

M

To ensure complete accuracy, frequent application of the appliance to the cast is necessary. If the foot was correctly reformed to its normal contours during the process of cast taking, the finished appliance should stand firmly on a flat surface without rocking. Any slight defect in this direction should be remedied. Care should be taken to grind and polish the edges of the metal in the concluding stages of processing (Fig. 71).

When fitting the appliance to the patient's foot, it should be clearly understood that correct functioning with the re-establishment of postural stability is not possible unless the footwear is suitable. It is not likely that any degree of success will be achieved with the Whitman brace if its use is attempted in conjunction with unsuitable footwear. The appliance must be able to seat itself and rest firm and stable on the insole of the shoe. The heel seat should be adequate to take the weightbearing heel, and the waist of the shoe should be sufficiently wide to accommodate the appliance. Proper width across the tread is also essential. In other words, a shoe with the correct heel-to-ball fitting, taking into account the appliance, is what is required. In the case of the Whitman brace, as in other corrective appliances of this nature, replacement is necessary at appropriate intervals when used in the treatment of children. Just as footwear has to be replaced to accommodate the growth and development of the child's foot, replacement and adjustment is necessary in the case of all forms of corrective surgical insoles.

Many modifications of the Whitman brace are made. For instance, the appliance is made with a heel seat and with the anterior portion of the appliance extending behind the heads of all the metatarsals as in the ordinary metal arch support.

It may be noted that, when processing the appliance, duraluminium needs more careful handling than either of the other metals when moulding the flange and clip, as it shows a greater tendency to fracture if any attempt is made to hurry the processing. Stainless steel may be used in gauge 16 with a fair degree of confidence, although gauge 20 is advocated in the case of malleable steel, and strongly advised when using duraluminium.

14

Shoe Therapy

I T is essential that the modern chiropodist should understand the basic principles of shoe construction and shoe fitting. It is particularly important that he should devote some time to the study of footwear in relation to children's feet. Many of the defects found in adults are the result of neglect in childhood. This does not necessarily imply that parents have been willingly negligent, but that proper advice and assistance were not available or the parents were not aware of such facilities.

A survey of school children carried out by the author, with the assistance of a team of senior students, during 1946 and 1947 produced some interesting facts. During the survey 5101 school children were examined, 20 schools being visited. Every child was examined for the following conditions:

> Defects of the longitudinal arch.
> Defects of the metatarsal arch.
> Lesser toe defects.
> Nail defects.
> Hallux valgus.
> Verrucæ pedis.
> Corns and callosities.

Footwear was examined and checked for size, fit and degree of serviceability. Three standards were set for each condition:

> 'A' for satisfactory,
> 'B' for slight defect, and
> 'C' for marked defect.

An analysis of the figures showed that the proportion of badly-fitting shoes in children entering school and children leaving school (about ten years later) averaged about the same. It should be noticed, however, that the incidence of defects in the feet was much higher in the older children, and that this applied to each type of defect. No children, on entering school, were found with serious defects of the metatarsal arch, or with nail conditions, verrucæ, corns or callosities. A few instances of slight congenital deformities of the lesser toes were recorded, but the number of such cases was negligible. Among the school-leavers, however, there was a very considerable incidence of all forms of defects. The proportion of slight and marked defects was approximately the same. Among the school-leavers corns and callosities were already in evidence. Corns and callosities showed an incidence of 11 per cent., whilst hallux valgus revealed an incidence of 26.4 per cent., and defects of the long arch were even higher. It is interesting to note the proportion of children with perfect feet at school-leaving was only half of those starting school, starters being 62.4 per cent. and leavers 33.4 per cent.

The collective figures on shoe fitting are most interesting. Children wearing shoes one size too small—girls 26.9 per cent., boys 22.3 per cent. Children wearing shoes at least two sizes too small—girls 10.3 per cent., boys 5.4 per cent. The collective figures show that approximately 34 per cent. of all children examined had footwear inaccurately fitted. A large proportion of toe defects were the direct result of ill-fitting footwear and tight hose. A recent investigation among adolescent secondary school children in a working-class district wearing footwear in sizes coming within the adult range (3 to 7) revealed an appallingly high percentage of severe defects of the lesser toes, advanced stages of pronated feet, and severe hallux valgus, whilst hallux rigidus with both early and advanced symptoms was encountered with disturbing frequency. Percentages are often misleading and must not be accepted as dogmatic indications of general proportions. Many factors tend to make percentages produced by survey misleading. If a survey is carried out at a school in which the children were drawn from a good social environment, it is found that the incidence of serious defects arising from footwear of unsuitable type is considerably less than in the case of children brought up in a bad social environment. It is found that many of the latter are wearing footwear of most unsuitable adult types, and in many instances wearing the parents' cast-off and trodden-over footwear. Nevertheless, making due allowance for such discrepancies, extensive and careful surveys carried out over long periods have established without question the fact that the most serious and permanent defects in children's feet are found to occur in disturbingly high percentages in the age group 12 to 16; 12 to 14 is included because the percentage in this sub-group is quite high, although it should be noticed that it is highest in the sub-group 14 to 16.

It has already been stated that in many cases defects in both feet and footwear are not the result of parental neglect, but lack of advice and assistance.

A chiropodist with the necessary knowledge can do much to assist in placing both child and adult in sound stabilising footwear. By this, it is not suggested that he should dabble in shoe retailing. The chiropodist can best help by examining the footwear being worn by the patient, pointing out any inaccuracies or defects in type or fitting, and give advice on the type of footwear best suited to the particular needs of the patient. Correctly designed footwear is fundamental in all shoe fitting. Footwear should conform to the physiological and anatomical principles of the human foot, and therefore in designing footwear the natural function and stability of the feet should be taken into account. Shoes should be designed to be complementary to these factors, exerting a corrective influence on feet showing structural and postural instability, whilst at the same time exerting no adverse effect on healthy feet.

In taking measurements to clothe the foot, it can generally be accepted that the girth measurement of the foot does not determine the internal capacity. The relative volume and shape is the real and essential factor. Mr Wm. J. Peake, writing in *The British Chiropody Journal*, October 1947, ably illustrates this point by the following diagrams:

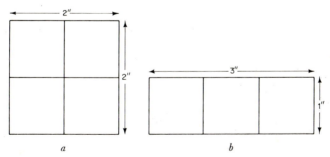

'It will readily be seen in the case of Fig. *a* that the outside measurement or girth of this perimeter is 8 inches, giving an internal capacity or area of 4 square inches. In Fig. *b* the outside measurement is still the same as in Fig. *a* (8 inches), but the internal capacity is only 3 square inches. The measurements of both perimeters are exactly the same, the areas are different. If these examples are exploited, it will be realised the variations that can be accomplished in footwear construction of any particular section, all measuring the same girth or external measurement, but giving different internal capacity. The nearer any section of the shoe gets to a circle the greater will be its internal capacity or volume. These examples are clear indication of the paramount importance of the distribution of the volume inside the shoe, or shape of the last upon which the shoe is made. The last model maker must acquire the intangible sense of size and form, the same sense which a sculptor possesses, combined with a structural knowledge of the foot.'

It is an understanding of this fundamental relationship between the foot form and the shoe, supported by an understanding of the basic principles of structural and postural stability, that provide the foundation upon which the chiropodist can build in the field of shoe therapy.

LEATHER

Origin of Leather

Leather was the first material used for the making of footwear, the skins of animals being scraped and stretched to cure them. When dried, they were made into simple, soft slippers by sewing them with sinews or thongs. The earliest method of preserving skins was to rub in grease and oils. The use of alum and the infusion of galls, vegetable matter and barks came much later. Sole leather was introduced into England by the Romans, who used oak bark in its manufacture. Leather dressing was probably introduced into Turkey by the Mohammedans, from whence these arts spread through Europe to England.

A Definition of Leather

Leather is an animal skin which has been preserved from natural decay by the use of fats, oils and a variety of chemical agents, after the loose, scaly epidermis and hair have been removed.

For the purpose of shoemaking, leather is the most suitable material ever produced. It possesses many valuable qualities. Not only is it strong, flexible and able to resist very severe friction and strain, but it is pliable, resilient, durable, light and, to a considerable degree, waterproof. No other material has been produced as a substitute that combines all the estimable qualities possessed by leather. Substitutes have, from time to time, been introduced for both uppers and soles. Rubber-impregnated materials have been tried as a substitute for leather, and recently plastics have been added to the list. All have proved very indifferent substitutes, and in many cases quite unsatisfactory. None could bear comparison with the original shoe-making material.

One of the primary defects in these substitutes is that they are non-porous. The natural excretions from the tissue cannot be absorbed by these materials, and as a result condensation occurs and a reabsorption of toxic substances by the tissues takes place. The condensation causes the skin to become moist and flaccid, resulting in maceration and blistering. The porosity, or ability to breathe, possessed by leather enables the waste products to escape by evaporation and absorption into the leather.

Whilst linen and cotton fabrics are porous, they are harsher to the skin and do not mould themselves to the form of the foot so well as leather, also repeated wetting and drying causes considerable shrinkage and distortion.

Enormous quantities of leather are used in this country in the making of boots and shoes. It has been authoritatively stated that over one hundred million pairs are manufactured in Britain every year, all made with uppers of leather.

Tanning

This term, which originally only applied to the preserving of skins by the use of tannic acid, is now used in a more liberal sense to embrace the processing of all leathers, the names of the various substances used being applied to distinguish them.

Types of Leathers

Almost any kind of skin can be made into leather. The skins of reptiles and even fish are made into leather, but only a limited range of animal skins are in ready demand, the commonest of these being the bull, cow, sheep and goat. Of the reptile skins, those of the crocodile, alligator and the lizard are most in demand. Whilst it is common practice to name the type of leather after the reptile from which it is made, in the case of animal skins a considerable variety of leathers are made from the same hide or skin. In the case of the ox, sole leather, leather for insoles and uppers are all processed from the same hide.

It should also be noted that different tanning and finishing methods produce leathers widely different in appearance from the same skin.

LASTS

Shoes are constructed on lasts which are the models, forms, or shapes over which the uppers are stretched, and determine the shape and cubic content of the shoe upon which they are made.

The bespoke boot-maker makes his boots and shoes on lasts which are made to measurements of his customers' own feet, and which faithfully reproduce their form and individual characteristics, whilst embodying such fundamentals as heel elevation, the raising of the heel of the last to accommodate the determined height of shoe heel and toe-spring. The old last-makers were highly skilled craftsmen, who were able to combine a native skill with the eye of an artist in shaping these wooden forms with wonderful accuracy.

In making lasts for mass-production shoes the last-maker works to fixed standards of measurements and sizes, which have been determined as the result of much research and investigation. It is generally claimed that these basic measurements are maintained irrespective of any variation in the shape of the last. This, in effect, means that the total volume of wood in a last of a certain size and fitting will be the same, although its displacement may vary in the production of different last shapes to accommodate various types of feet.

As hard pavements require modern shoes to have strong insulating soles which are relatively stiff, heels are introduced to assist in the take-off and also absorb some of the shock of impact in walking.

The two extreme positions of the foot when walking are (a) when the heel contacts the ground, and (b) when the toes leave the ground in the last act of propulsion. As stock shoes made for either of these extreme positions would not be satisfactory, a position between the two extremes is determined and is arrived at by designing the last to take a heel and by raising the toe of the last. The latter is termed toe-spring. These two factors assist in the take-off in walking.

Whilst lasts have recently been made of other materials, they are generally made from wood. A variety of hard woods are used, but lasts made from maple or hemlock are said to be the best. Great care is taken in drying and seasoning the wood. Kiln-drying is resorted to to prevent any possibility of shrinkage and warping after the lasts are made.

It has already been stated that the various sizes and widths are developed from basic measurements, and are then produced in basic models. All sizes and fittings are graded from these. Most manufacturers use three basic models, sizes 4, 6 and 8, with two or even three widths in each size.

MEASUREMENTS

In measuring the foot we may be doing so with a view to making a pair of shoes, or with the object of building up a set of patterns for use in mass-production shoemaking. It cannot be stressed too much that the strictest accuracy is necessary. The graduation in sizes is extremely small, and in consequence even a fraction of variation in measurement is of great importance.

The foot is usually measured at the following points, viz. joint, waist, instep, heel and ankle. The instep measurement may be supplemented by the Hass measure, which is sometimes termed the high instep. The heel measurement is taken at two points, one measurement is termed the long heel and the other the short heel. The ankle measurement is taken just above the ankle joint (Fig. 72).

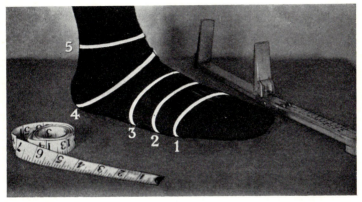

FIG. 72

Showing the principal measurements, size stick and tape measure.

1. Joint measurement.   3. Instep measurement.
2. Waist measurement.   4. Heel measurement.
                           5. Ankle measurement.

Joint Measurement

The joint measurement is very important, and requires very careful application. Various types of feet will show a considerable variation in the angulation of the hinge formed by the metatarso-phalangeal joints. In some feet it will be noted that the hinge is almost transverse, whilst in others it will be markedly oblique. The measurement is taken round the widest points on the first and fifth metatarsal heads.

Waist Measurement

This measurement is taken immediately behind the first and fifth metatarso-phalangeal joints, and should be the smallest possible measurement that can be taken at this point.

Instep Measurement

Two forms of instep measurement are in common use, one is to measure one-half of the length of the foot from the back of the heel, corresponding in height with the top of the instep. This gives the point at which the girth of the instep is measured. Another method is to take the measurement from a point located at the prominence of the internal cuniform bone.

Hass Measurement

This measurement, not often used nowadays except by a few old craftsmen, is taken round the instep over the posterior aspect of the navicular, and posterior to the cuboid.

Long-Heel Measurement

This is another measurement that is now little used. It is taken round a central point on the ball of the heel and over the prominence on the internal cuniform.

Heel Measurement

The heel measurement should be very carefully taken from the ball of the heel round the throat curve, which is the point anterior to the ankle joint, and at which it bends in dorsiflexion of the foot.

Ankle Measurement

It has already been explained that this measurement is taken round the leg just above the ankle joint.

Leg Measurement

These measurements are always taken at carefully gauged distances up the leg from the base of the heel, and when quoted the measurement up the leg should also be given, along with the girth measurement at that point.

Bespoke Shoes

Whilst the measurements just described are used in designing basic models from which the lasts for mass-production shoes are made, such measurements are also used in the designing of the individual lasts in bespoke shoe-making.

As the old craftsmen have died out, the art of making these lasts has also gradually become almost forgotten, and in recent years most bespoke shoe-makers have resorted to the modifying of stock lasts to their customers' measurements, unless the defects in the feet amounted to severe deformities. When the modifications required are excessive the alteration of stock lasts is out of the question. In this event, casts of the patient's feet are usually sent up to the last maker so that a special pair of lasts may be made to the required form and measurements. For many years the author used stock lasts of this type as a basis for designing lasts to the measurements of his patients' feet. The technique was to use lasts of a suitable shape and pitch, but much oversize so as to provide ample volume of spare wood upon which to work. With measurements, drafts marked with both dorsal and plantar defects, contour drawings and casts the lasts were reduced to the proper shape and measurements by using the scouring wheels on a shoe finishing machine, rasps, sandpaper, etc. Occasionally plastic wood or leather was resorted to for very local adjustments. These lasts, which became the property of the patient, proved a boon to a great many of them, and footwear made on these lasts proved a major contribution to successful treatment.

Specials

Many of the high-grade shoe manufacturers provide a special service for their customers or agents. This service consists of modified stock lasts to measurements submitted and the making of special shoes upon these lasts. The shoe retailer selects a size, shape and fitting from stock as near as possible to the requirements of his customer. The next step is to take drafts, marking any defects such as dorsal and distal corns, bunions, exostoses, etc.

The feet are now measured; a modification of the full range of measurements is used, usually shoe size, ball, instep and heel only being taken, except when boots are required, in which case the ankle measurements are given. This system has proved very beneficial to many foot sufferers, and it is most desirable that some form of liaison between the shoe retailer and the orthopædist or chiropodist should be established whereby footwear requiring only minor alterations could be made in this way without resorting to the fully-fledged bespoke shoes.

This system is particularly useful for women patients as the appearance of such shoes are invariably more presentable than bespoke shoes. It should, however, be remembered that this system is only useful when minor alterations will meet the case, such as a little fitting on a joint, a little more depth for the toes, generally, or over a hammer toe in particular. The curvature of the long arch may be increased by scouring out the required amount of wood, but care has to be taken to retain the correct girth measurement of the instep by adding new material in the form of plastic wood or leather to the top of the last when necessary.

THE FOOTWEAR OF THE CHILD

It is believed by many that all children are born with perfect feet, which are subsequently distorted and weakened by footwear. This is a false assumption. Some children are born with structural defects, and most children in a civilized community have feet that pronate to some degree when standing. If the child born with sound, healthy feet could be kept without shoes and brought up in an environment of springy turf and soft sand during the pre-school years, structural and postural stability would be assured, provided that on beginning to wear shoes they were based upon sound anatomical and physiological principles. As the modern child usually commences active life in the environment of unyielding wooden floors and later hard, stony or concrete pavements, development of the intrinsic muscles is retarded. As these conditions are part and parcel of a civilized existence, it is a practical policy to assist the child in developing sound, modern feet by fitting appropriate footwear at an early age to assist in establishing and retaining structural and postural stability. If this principle is accepted, it will be agreed that the best time to fit the child with appropriate footwear is when the first steps are taken towards assuming an erect posture.

The efficiency of the modern foot is dependent on its ability to act effectively as a lever, and its efficient functioning in this capacity is dependent on a semi-rigid tarsus and a sound and massive first metatarsal segment.

If we are to accept the modern foot with its more or less rigid tarsus as a normal standard, footwear with a flexible shank cannot be approved. A sound shoe for a child is one which firmly supports the tarsus. Such a shoe requires a rigid shank and adequate length to accommodate the growing foot. The shoe should be based on a fitting from heel to ball. This means that the waist of the shoe should fit snugly under the instep to immediately behind the heads of the metatarsal joints.

The stability of the first metatarsal segment is impaired by any of the common anomalies which affect the first metatarsal bone (i.e. shortness, hypermobility or varus inclination), so that the anterior medial corner of the foot tripod is weakened and the foot tends to pronate. Sound footwear should take account of this tendency and should ensure the effective positioning of the first metatarsal segment in the shoe so that a postural stability is established.

The Heel-to-Ball Fitting

By this system shoes are fitted to the arch length. The foot is measured on a scale in which the shoe size coincides with the level of the ball joint. In this method of shoe fitting the shoe length from heel to ball coincides with the foot length over this area, the joint resting in the widest part of the shoe, and the metatarso-phalangeal joints or the hinge of the foot coincide with the hinge part of the shoe (Fig. 73).

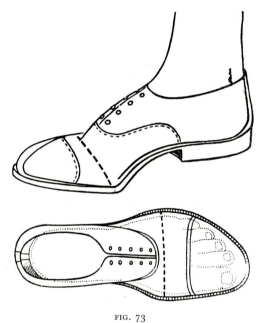

FIG. 73

Illustration showing transparent view through shoe of the relationship between the hinge of the foot and shoe.

In this form of fitting, toe length is taken into account, and is provided for in the fitting range. Adequate length and joint fitting are essential, because on weightbearing some degree of lengthening of the foot takes place, with a degree of spreading across the metatarso-phalangeal area. Short shoes will cause injury to nails, whilst back pressure on the end of the great toe can seriously damage the first metatarso-phalangeal joint. Shoes which are too narrow across the tread will cramp the foot and impair muscle function, leading to loss of muscle tonus and atrophy.

The shoe should be closely tailored around the heel and the instep. The heel fitting should be close and snug, including the corseting of the sub-taloid joint (Fig. 74). Whilst the shoe should fit closely round the heel and instep, there should be full and ample joint fitting and complete freedom for the toes so as to allow, as far as is possible in footwear (Figs 75 *a* and *b*), a satisfactory positioning of the first metatarsal segment, and the maintenance of postural stability. As the foot of the child has not yet been distorted by shoes, every endeavour should be made to clothe the foot in shoes that conform to the natural contours.

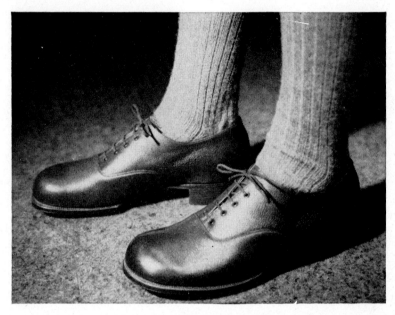

FIG. 74
These shoes are correct at the joint instep, heel and ankle.
By courtesy of British Boot, Shoe, and Allied Trades Research Association.

A child's foot differs from that of the adult in its anatomical development. In the child's foot there is considerable spacing between the articulations of the joints, and in a very young child there is a lagging in the development of the mid-tarsal segment in relation to the rest of the foot structure. Because of these factors, it is very easy to fit a child with a shoe that is very much too short without the child actually suffering pain. The greatest care should therefore be taken to see that adequate length is provided (Fig. 76). By most

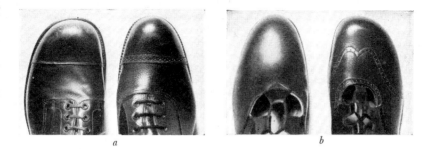

FIG. 75
Toe shape.

a. For Boys.
A good shape. A bad shape.

b. For Girls.
A bad shape. A good one.

By courtesy of British Boot, Shoe, and Allied Trades Research Association.

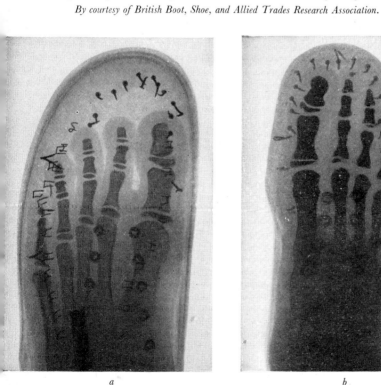
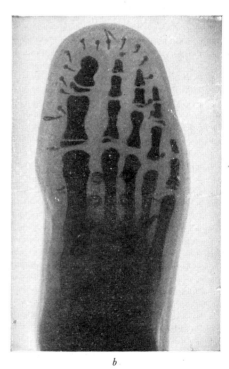

a

b

FIG. 76
Showing toe line in relation to the shoe.

a. Correct length.

b. Too short.

By courtesy of British Boot, Shoe, and Allied Trades Research Association.

authorities adequate length means $\frac{3}{4}$ inch beyond the length of the longest toe. The term 'longest toe' is used because there are many cases in which the longest toe is not necessarily the great toe. When a child is firmly established on its feet, the toe extension may be reduced to $\frac{1}{2}$ inch, as excessive extension may do more harm than good, leading to faulty gait and imbalance. It is also essential that measurements should be taken with the feet weightbearing, and standing with them 6 inches apart. Measurements taken in this way allow for hypermobility and extension.

Children outgrow their shoes within four to five months, and it is therefore advisable that systematic checking of the foot measurements in relation to shoe size should be carried out at regular intervals of not more than three months (Fig. 77).

In clothing the foot of the young child, that is a child up to about $2\frac{1}{2}$ years of age, boots rather than shoes are advisable. This is not advocated, as some might think, to support the weak ankles, but because the mobility of the joints and the simple architecture of the foot of a very young child make it difficult to keep a low shoe on the foot, let alone retain it in close proximity to the instep and ankle, providing the stabilising support that is necessary. It is the boot rather than the shoe that can be most successfully secured on a child's foot. Dr H. R. Tax in his book *Podopediatrics* ably disposes of the weak ankle theory for boots by stating ankle motion is of a hinge joint variety and its principal motion is flexion and extension. The so-called 'weak ankle' or 'double ankle' is not weak ankle at all, but a weakness of the foot called pronation. This movement (pronation) consists of a rolling inwards and downwards of the foot, and takes place at the sub-taloid joint which lies below the ankle. Most Oxford shoes are so built that they cover this joint completely, giving it support. The need for the higher shoe, therefore, is not at all one for added support for the foot. Support for the foot is directly dependent on the bottom and inner border of the shoe, and the Oxford (low shoe) fills this requirement as well as the boot.

It is to retain the bottom and inner border in close proximity to the foot in the very young child that boots rather than shoes are advocated. After the child has reached $2\frac{1}{2}$ years of age, however, shoes may be introduced as a satisfactory form of footwear.

Rigid Shank

Reference has already been made to the importance of the rigid shank in the shoe which clothes and supports the modern foot. Unlike the primitive foot, which was a more flexible and mobile

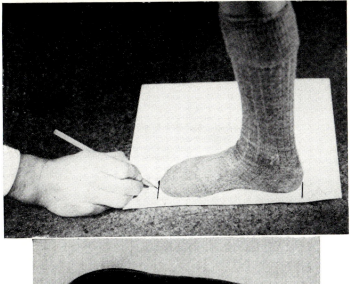

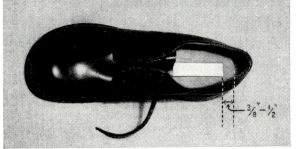

FIG. 77

Checking the length of a shoe.

To make sure the shoes have not become too short, have the child stand barefoot on a piece of cardboard. With a pencil put one mark at the end of the longest toe and another at the back of the heel. Cut out a strip of the cardboard about ½ inch wide, between the two marks. Insert the strip in the inside of the shoe and when one end of it is pushed up to the toe, the other end should be at least ⅜ inch to ½ inch short of the back of the shoe.

By courtesy of British Boot, Shoe, and Allied Trades Research Association.

structure, the modern foot has of necessity become more compact, and the tarsus more rigid to form an efficient lever. The limitation in adduction of the great toe and first metatarsal segment in shoes and hose results in a narrowing of the base of the triangle of stability.

In this way the most important prop of the medial arch is weakened, and a rigid shank is necessary to provide some compensatory if inadequate support.

We must always have in the forefront of our minds the fact that

N

the child is in the unnatural environment of hard, unyielding floor surfaces, as against the ideal one of springy turf, soft sand, etc.

Whilst the waist of the shoe should be stiffened by the use of the rigid shank, the hinge movement of the metatarso-phalangeal joints should be accommodated by a flexible sole that bends truly at this point.

FOOTWEAR OF THE ADULT

In approaching the subject of adult footwear, one has to consider feet which are mature, having assumed their final form and characteristics; also, in the great majority of cases permanent structural defects have to be taken into account.

It will be found on careful study that the feet can be classified and placed into various type groups, whilst functional classification is also not only possible but very necessary. The classification of feet in this way plays a vital part in the scientific fitting of shoes. In fact, it is the object of the expert shoe fitter to select and fit footwear of a type suited to the form and functional type of the customer. The chiropodist may not be selecting and fitting the actual shoes for his patient, but it is of very great importance that he is able to recognise the characteristics of his patient's feet, and accurately assess the degree to which the footwear does or does not measure up to requirements.

It is already acknowledged that a great proportion of minor deformities are acquired as the result of wearing ill-fitting footwear over a long period of time. Whilst in many cases the patient has not been aware of any discomfort associated with the abnormality or deformity, he is painfully conscious of secondary lesions due to postural instability arising from deformity.

Foot Types

It is most interesting and instructive to study our patients' feet, not only as a means of diagnosing lesions and abnormalities but as a means of classifying them into the various types and functional classes.

In the course of our study we shall observe the long narrow foot, often with the toes falling away at a very oblique angle from the second to the fifth. This type of foot is frequently thin, with only a limited amount of padding. We may then observe what is often erroneously regarded as the normal foot, with its pleasing lines and apparent good balance between length and joint width, and the nice curve of the toe line as it falls gradually away from a second that is slightly longer than the first to the fifth toe. In due course we will be sure to encounter the short plump foot. This foot is short, broad and well padded. The tips of the toes are usually set in an almost straight line from the great toe to the fifth.

These are three basic types that are regularly encountered, variation in degree will, of course, be found in each type, but the basic types are as such easily recognised. We will meet a varying degree of arch elevation, from a medial arch with a very pronounced curve to a foot in which the arch is very shallow. These variations in character are testimony of the fact that we each and every one of us individually possess distinct features of form and character.

The various factors described in relation to the different foot types are merely features of the individual. All are normal unless some development occurs that impairs function—all such developments may be classified as abnormal.

Function

Having considered foot types, we must consider function and classify feet accordingly. We have the flaccid or hypermobile foot which on weightbearing flows in all directions. This type of foot has a very great degree of flexibility. We have the type of foot which has a degree of flexibility that provides for an adequate degree of movement, but its range of flexibility is not exaggerated. This again is the type that we are apt to regard as the normal. Again, we can classify a further type that may be termed rigid: this type has an extremely limited range of movement. We may meet this condition in the obese oedematous type or in the thin bony foot associated with senile degeneration.

It has long been realised that when advocating the heel-to-ball fitting system for shoes, anomalies did exist which when met with would militate against a satisfactory fit. The abnormally long second or fourth metatarsal are examples that are encountered from time to time. It is found that in such cases the hinge movement of the shoe across the tread in a line from the first to fifth metatarsal is impaired, and so brings excessive friction and pressure to bear upon the prominent metatarsal, which is depressed by back pressure on the end of the toe in many cases.

A factor that is important is that of the tight tendo Achillis, a condition that may be congenital or acquired. The wearing of very high heels over a prolonged period of time will produce the objective symptoms of short tendo Achillis, although the condition is more frequently one of shortening of the calf muscles. In such cases the patient will have no difficulty in carrying out a normal range of movement in plantar flexion, but it will be found that the range of dorsiflexion is very limited or entirely absent, the patient being unable to move this foot beyond a position at right-angles to the leg. This case has its own special problems to be dealt with when fitting shoes. The acquired short tendo Achillis is almost invariably a defect of women, although the congenital condition is met with in males.

Flare Factors

When referring to 'flare' we mean the in-swerve or out-swerve of the forefoot as a design characteristic.

The question of relationship of flare of feet and shoes has come into considerable prominence of recent years, and much thought has been expended on this factor by many orthopædic surgeons, chiropodists and shoe fitters. It must be conceded that in the main natural feet have a tendency to in-flare, whilst a degree of pronation will induce valgus deviation of the forefoot, which may in consequence be classified as an out-flare foot. Between these two deviations we have the foot that is straight.

In the case of the middle-aged or elderly adult, a valgus forefoot will not be easily corrected, and the out-flare tendency has to be taken into account. As most adults have acquired quite a reasonable degree of hallux valgus, the in-flare factor will seldom arise. A study of the foot of the adult, particularly the feet of women, will reveal the fact that the forefoot of many have assumed a conical form due to the wearing of tight hose or shoes of that shape, and here we are brought back to the straight shoe. The straight foot and out-flare foot are in the main the result of acquired deformity or weakness. The in-flare foot, unless deviated to the degree of a deformity, is the somewhat rare case in the adult, an approach to the natural foot. It is important that these tendencies be noted and taken into account in shoe fitting (Fig. 78).

Classification of foot types should not be concluded without some reference to the relationship of heel and joint. Whilst many feet show a relationship of heel and joint size that conforms to the average of fittings carried by the shoe store, a considerable number of feet are encountered with a narrow heel and a wide joint. Feet of this type require equal care in the fitting of the heel as of the joint, if the shoe is to remain comfortable and the foot retained properly seated in the heel of the shoe. The foot with a wide heel and narrow joint is a much rarer type, but it is equally important that special consideration should be given to the heel fitting.

An effort has been made to provide a limited range of heel fittings, as well as joint fittings, in mass-produced shoes of good makes, but a full range carried by retail shoe stores would involve a considerable outlay in stock, much of which in the case of the fittings in little demand means an appreciable amount of capital locked up in stock with a very slow turnover. The result is that the retailer is tempted to carry only a skeleton range, with the object of fitting the majority from stock and ordering the special fittings as required.

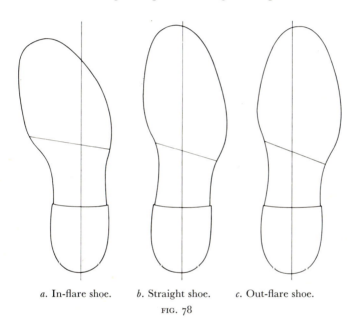

a. In-flare shoe.   b. Straight shoe.   c. Out-flare shoe.

FIG. 78

THE SIGNIFICANCE OF WEAR MARKS ON FOOTWEAR

In addition to careful case-taking and observation of the patient, attention should be paid to the patterns of wear on the patient's shoes. Much has been said and written about the part played by ill-fitting footwear in bringing about deformities, painful lesions and excrescences, but less has been said about the effect of defective feet upon the footwear.

Feet that are unstable as the result of painful pressure areas, excrescences and congenital or acquired deformities will bring to bear stresses upon the footwear, producing distortion and abnormal wear that will provide the experienced practitioner with a wealth of information.

The accurate interpretation of wear marks and other abnormal features will make a valuable contribution to the accumulated evidence that will enable an accurate diagnosis to be made.

We should consider the wear marks under three headings, namely those resulting from the normal wear of healthy feet in good-fitting footwear, variations from the normal due to ill-fitting footwear and, finally, abnormal wear marks brought about by changes in gait being a manifestation of foot trouble.

Normal Walking

Healthy feet properly stabilised in footwear that has been correctly fitted show wear marks that are fairly evenly distributed. There will be slight wearing away at the toes, a more pronounced wearing across the tread and across the back of the heel. The wear mark on the heel will be slightly off-centre towards the outside (Fig. 79). Another factor which will be noted is that in an accurately fitted shoe the flexure creases across the vamp situated in the depression at the base of the toes and the upper will, at no point, overhang the edge of the sole.

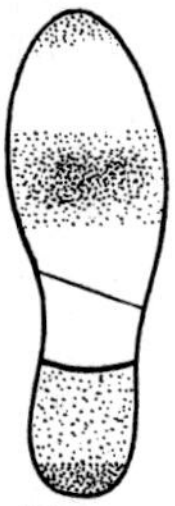

FIG. 79

Area of sole and heel wear from a normal foot, showing areas of greatest concentration.

If one examines the insole of the shoe one will see that the imprint of the foot is evenly distributed with no deep depressions. Also there will be no particular wear marks observed on the heel counter.

Signs of Faulty Fitting

When shoes have been fitted short, the toes will make an impression in the toe-box. In some cases, the toe-cap will be pushed forward. The point of the impingement of the great toe-nail is sometimes seen as a slight bulge at this point, while if one places one's fingers on the inside of the toe-box, one will be able to feel where the nail cuts deeply into it. The back pressure on the heel will also exhibit its signs in the form of excessive wear on the linings of the quarters on either side of the heel counter. A tight, short shoe prevents the normal free function of the foot when walking, the foot being held almost rigid. Excessive wear will be found at the tip of the toe and the back of the heel. Often the vamp will be found to show excessive fullness and in the open tab or derby type of shoe it will be found that they do not lace sufficiently closely. This is particularly so if the shoes have an inadequate amount of room in the fitting as well as in the length. The shoes may well also gape at the ankle, when bending the foot.

In many cases, shoes for the middle-aged women are made on lasts with a conical toe with extra fitting at the joint in an endeavour to accommodate the enlargement caused by an exostosis. With the desire to give the shoes an appearance of lightness the soles are often made with a pump-edge finish, dispensing with a welt. The misplacement of the additional accommodation dorsally instead of laterally on the great toe joint results in the exostosis forcing the upper out to the side, resulting in some unsightly creasing and a marked treading over at this point. Also the excessive pressure on the lining over the exostosis causes it to be quickly worn through. In the endeavour to produce the illusion of lightness and slimness, the waist of the shoe is also usually too narrow with the result that the foot overhangs onto the upper, pressing down upon it and causing gaping at the ankle.

Another fault in shoe fitting which is frequently encountered is one in which a shoe has been fitted with too small a heel seat. As the heel does not seat properly in the shoe it slips badly when walking, the stockings wear at the heel and blistering at the heel frequently occurs owing to the considerable friction. The margin of the heel becomes very tender and the skin becomes thick and calloused. Sometimes a blister underlies the callous tissue. Friction and tenderness are very severe if the heel counter is a strong one. If the heel counter is weak, however, the heel of the foot will force it out over the face of the shoe heel exposing the edge of the insole at the heel. The heel of the foot will tend to overhang this on weightbearing as it forces the counter outwards, thus exposing it to further irritation and much discomfort.

In many high-heeled shoes, the heel seat does not lie parallel with the sole but forms a continuous slope with the waist. As a result the foot in use is precipitated down this sloping platform into the forepart of the shoe causing excessive back pressure on the toes as they are forced into the toe-box. The weight distribution of the body through the foot is interfered with, causing it to be directed forward onto the ball of the foot, resulting in excessive pressure at this point. This condition is further aggravated by the extreme angulation of the toes through back pressure.

The effect on the shoe will be seen in the great tension across the vamp which will be trodden over the margin of the sole. The mark of the excessive pressure will be shown in the ball of the shoe by staining from excessive perspiration and the retracted toes cause the inter-phalangeal joints to be forced into the upper producing bulges where they make permanent impressions.

If the high-heeled shoe is to avoid these pitfalls the heel seat should be horizontal and on the same plane as the sole although at a higher level. In court shoes the tendency to slide forward frequently causes the edge of the vamp to cut into the foot resulting in much discomfort and dorsal oedema.

Foot Defects

Wear marks reflect almost every kind of foot trouble. The experienced practitioner will study these and by them be able to confirm his diagnosis or be assisted in arriving at one.

Long Arch Weakness

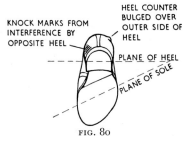

FIG. 80

Twist between sole and heel occurring as a result of mobile foot strain.

In long arch weakness wear marks vary according to whether or not the feet abduct on weightbearing. Should the feet abduct the shoes will be found to be worn down on the posterior-lateral border of the heels and on the innerside of the soles. This causes the shoes to develop a twist between the soles and the heels (Fig. 80).

If you were to stand the shoes on a table it would be seen that they rock slightly from side to side. This indication of instability is due to the twist which is caused by abduction brought about by the feet rolling inwards causing a tilting of the heels into eversion. This results in an angular thrust at the outer base of the heel counters. Not only are the heels worn over on the outer side but often the heel counters are caused to bulge over.

The feet being in an abducted position causes the posterior lateral area of the shoe heels to strike the ground at each step. This ultimately causes excessive wear, further undermining stability and causing an increase in the bulge at the heel counter. Where the heels turn over on the outer border into a forced inversion, even though the former position was that of eversion, the higher the heel and the smaller the top-piece, the more readily will this reaction be induced.

A tight tendo Achilles can also be responsible for abducting a mobile pronated foot and one should therefore give consideration to this possibility (Fig. 81*a*). This abduction is indicated by 'knock marks' which are abrasions on the shoe heels caused by the striking of each other as they pass in the process of walking and brought about by the inclination of the heels towards each other. If the abduction is not very severe the inward roll of the foot causes excessive wear on the inner border of the sole and heel. It is usually the inner front corner of the heel which is affected and the waist of the shoe is also broken down (Fig. 81*b*).

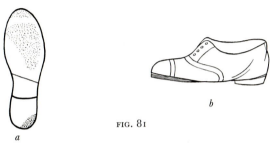

FIG. 81

a. Area of sole and heel wear in weak foot (mobile foot strain). *b.* Medial view of shoe in severe weak foot.

If the shoes are stood side by side they will be found to lean markedly inwards and they will bulge away from the ankles at the quarters. The uppers overhang along the outer border from the heel to the toe. Where the vamp and quarters meet under the arch of the foot there will be a long shallow bulge and also a shallow

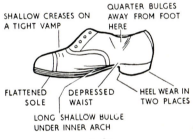

FIG. 82

The wear marks in chronic flat foot.

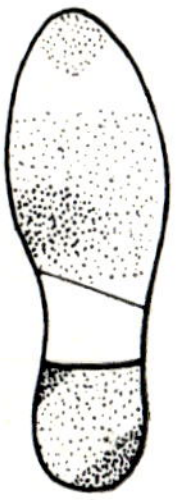

crease across the vamps. Impressions will have been made on the lateral inside of the toe-box while impressions of the metatarsal heads on the insoles will be clearly seen. In the condition usually referred to as chronic flat foot, in addition to the wearing away of the inner corner of the heel, the breast of the heel will have pressed deeply into the waist causing a buckling at the point where it meets, with the waist bulging downwards and the sole and waist becoming almost level (Figs 82–83).

FIG. 83

Area of sole and heel wear in chronic rigid flat foot showing greatest concentration at opposite corners of the heel and extension from sole back toward waist.

Metatarsalgia and Splay Foot

A splaying out of the forefoot causing a stretching of the vamp very

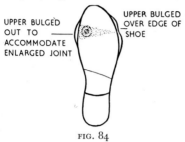

UPPER BULGED OUT TO ACCOMMODATE ENLARGED JOINT

UPPER BULGED OVER EDGE OF SHOE

FIG. 84

Area of sole wear in metatarsalgia with second hammer toe and non-rigid hallux valgus.

tightly, with considerable impingement upon the first and the fifth metatarsal joints, invariably results in overhang of the sole across the whole of the forefoot at both sides. Symptoms of metatarsalgia with the feet hot and burning cause considerable discoloration on the insole of the shoe in which there are deep impressions across the tread (Fig. 84).

Pes Cavus

This is a more or less rigid type of foot. There is a deep impression across the tread (metatarsal area), the toes are retracted and the sole is curved like a rocker. There will be considerable creasing across the vamp at the base of the toes. Across the tread at the point of greatest pressure the upper will overhang the sole. There is also considerable pressure in the heel seat. The heel usually splays out, causing wear on the heel counter with signs of considerable pressure. The patient usually has metatarsal callosities and callousing round the margin of the heel due to friction and pressure. There is heavy wear at the back of the shoe heel and across the sole at the tread (Fig. 85).

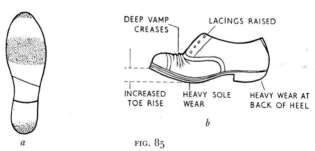

DEEP VAMP CREASES   LACINGS RAISED

INCREASED TOE RISE   HEAVY SOLE WEAR   HEAVY WEAR AT BACK OF HEEL

b

a   FIG. 85

a. Area of sole and heel wear in pes cavus. *b*. The wear marks of pes cavus.

Hallus Valgus

The valgus deviation of the great toe makes the joint stand out very prominently and as there is frequently a considerable exostosis and even a distended bursa, there is a considerable bulge and the shoe

upper is forced out. The upper overhangs the sole very considerably at
this point. There are frequently
ugly creases across the vamp and
very considerable wear on the ball
of the great toe joint (Fig. 86).

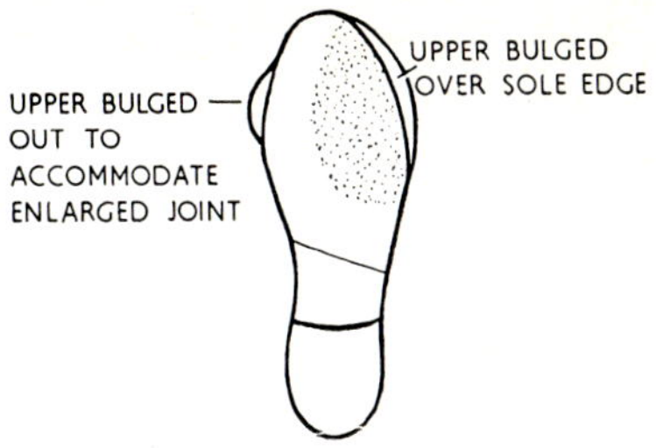

UPPER BULGED —
OUT TO
ACCOMMODATE
ENLARGED JOINT

UPPER BULGED
OVER SOLE EDGE

FIG. 86

Area of sole wear in rigid hallux valgus.

Hallux Rigidus

In this condition the shoe upper is usually tight over the dorsal
aspect of the joint with marked creasing of the upper forward of it.
Owing to the lack of movement in the metatarso-phalangeal joint,
it is transferred forward to the inter-phalangeal joint causing the
sole to be sharply angulated at this point, hence the ugly creasing
of the upper over this area. Usually a very painful callosity is
developed beneath the inter-phalangeal joint due to its unusual
responsibility. Great stress at this point frequently results in a bursting away of the welt.

In hallus rigidus the wear marks are found to be beneath the
distal joint on the inner side and beneath the fifth metatarsal joint
on the outer side. Whilst the greatest wear will be at this point,
excessive wear will take place all along the outer side of the sole as
the foot is thrown over to this side in an unconscious movement to
avoid using the painful great toe joint. This also causes a bulging of
the upper over the sole in this area (Fig. 87).

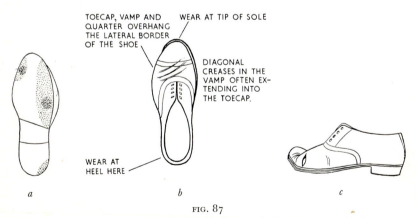

TOECAP, VAMP AND
QUARTER OVERHANG
THE LATERAL BORDER
OF THE SHOE

WEAR AT TIP OF SOLE

DIAGONAL
CREASES IN THE
VAMP OFTEN EX-
TENDING INTO
THE TOECAP.

WEAR AT
HEEL HERE

a   b   c

FIG. 87

a. Sole view of wear marks of hallux rigidus. b. The wear marks of hallux
rigidus. c. Sole upturned at level of inter-phalangeal joint.

SHOE FITTING

In measuring the foot for stock shoes the measurement should be taken while weightbearing. The reason for this is to provide for the natural spread of the foot when weight is placed upon it, whilst elongation to some degree will be encountered. The instrument used for this purpose is a standard size stick, which is a boxwood rule marked off in sizes and half-sizes from infant's to men's. At the base of this size stick is a stop against which the back of the heel will rest, another stop is fitted with a metal clip fixing it onto the stick, but permitting it to slide freely up and down.

To take the measure, the foot is placed on the size stick with the heel against the fixed stop. The movable one is moved along the stick until it is touching the great toe, except in cases where the great toe is not the longest, and then it should rest against the longest toe. Cases are met with where the second toe is the longest, and in much rarer cases another of the lesser toes. Such cases, of course, complicate the process of fitting shoes.

In the last design, allowance is made for a reasonable toe clearance which is about the equivalent to two sizes over the actual foot size. It is therefore necessary to allow two sizes over the size shown on the measure when the foot measurement is taken. Some manufacturers design size sticks with the required allowance provided, but in such cases this measuring instrument will only be reliable when used in conjunction with the makers' own shoes. Frequently manufacturers design a special range of lasts and size gradings accompanied by a measuring system requiring a special machine, which they have designed expressly for the purpose of accurately incorporating the foot measurement into the particular size and fitting required in their own particular range of shoes. No objection can be taken to this method of fitting stock shoes, provided the use of the measuring instrument is confined to the fitting of the particular footwear for which it was designed. The heel-to-ball principle of shoe fitting can be taken as being accepted as the most satisfactory standard method. Certain principles should be followed out in the fitting of shoes which can always be applied irrespective of any variety of fitting systems.

Adequate allowance should be made for the foot when weight-bearing to have ample length for toe clearance. Sufficient depth in the toe-box is also necessary. This point is most important when the toe tends to hyperextend. Another important point is to see that the heel-to-ball fitting of the shoe is correct. The heads of the metatarsals should seat accurately on the hinge of the shoe sole when the heel of the foot is placed snugly back into the heel of the shoe. The joint fit should be such as not to constrict the foot on weightbearing, whilst not allowing undue surplus material across the vamp to form creases. When laced, the fastening should tend to hold the foot back into the heel seat of the shoe. The upper should lace evenly and should not quite meet when properly fastened. When laced, the shoe should feel to corset and brace the instep and clip snugly round the heel, and the shoe should have been made on a last that conforms as near as possible to the foot type of the patient.

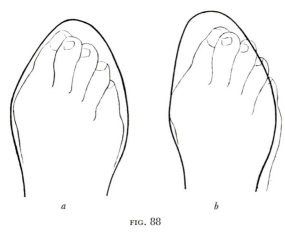

a   *b*

FIG. 88

a. Outline of shoe properly related to the grossly deformed foot. *b.* Outline of natural form shoe over the grossly deformed foot.

Shoes made on the straight-inside edge principle should be approached with caution in the case of the adult. The straight-inside edge last is really a fully in-flared shoe based on the natural foot, and few adult feet will be found to conform to the shape of this last. A modification of this type of shoe is also made with a slight outward deviation from the centre line which will, in consequence, fit a correspondingly greater number of adults. It will be found that in the great majority of cases the best shaped shoe is one in which the medial line of the forepart of the shoe deviates outwards to a noticeable degree, and in which the lateral curve follows a normal toe line; in other words, a shoe that is just short of being an out-flare shoe. The reason that a last of this type is suggested as conforming to the requirements of the greater number is that surveys have shown that in the average adult foot the anterior metatarsal area has spread but the toes have been retained in a more or less crowded position. Correction is not as a rule very hopeful, but adequate accommodation for the foot, as it is, frequently proves the best line of approach. Many chiropodists have met patients with a gross valgus deviation of the great toe with a considerable exostosis, yet the joint was freely movable, and no discomfort experienced unless the joint was impinged upon. Patients are met with who have burrowing fifth toes, in which the same principle applies. It is, in the opinion of the writer, a much sounder policy to treat such feet by prescribing shoes that fit snugly round the heel and instep, giving a firm bracing effect, whilst using a last with a forepart shape that allows adequate room for the joints and toes, yet conforming reasonably accurately to the shape of the foot. The fitting of adult feet requires the application of a great amount of common sense (Fig. 88).

Instances have come to the notice of the writer where the practitioner has endeavoured to apply corrective treatment to a case of hallux valgus with chronic bunion by the fitting of a shoe made on a straight-inside edge last. Needless to say that as a corrective treatment the fitting of such shoes was a dismal failure. Hallux valgus in a middle-aged person has come to stay, likewise the exostosis accompanying the chronic bunion. In the shoe referred to, the toe still retained its valgus deviation, leaving an empty space on the medial side of the toe-box and vamp which quickly resulted in an ugly crease on walking and caused an abrasion on the dorsal aspect of the proximal phalanx of the great toe. The valgus displacement of the toe causes a like tendency in the lesser toes, resulting in a severe impingement on the fourth toe by the lateral border of this in-flare shoe.

Bunion Shoe

The common-sense and more successful line of approach would have been to fit a bunion shoe. This type of shoe was first made on the assumption that the big joint fitting required corresponding roominess elsewhere. It was soon realised, however, that when a shoe was fitted that did not snugly embrace the instep and heel, the foot tended to creep forward in the shoe during wear. This resulted in a crowding into the fore part and an aggravation of the existing defects. The lesser toes were forced back and the valgus deviation of the great toe increased. The enforced subluxation of the metatarso-phalangeal joints usually induced symptoms of metatarsalgia. It is now realised that the patient with metatarsal spread and a chronic bunion frequently requires a small heel fitting, and shoes of this type are now produced. The bunion shoe properly fitted would conform reasonably well to the form of the foot and accommodate the joint. If a snug heel and instep fitting is achieved, the result will be real comfort for the patient. Correction will not result, but this is rarely possible in such cases except by surgery, and a worsening of the structural defects will be arrested, while the absence of any impingement will render the bunion more amenable to treatment if inflammation is present.

THE RELATIONSHIP OF HEEL AND LAST

The heel, provided that it is of modest height, plays a useful part under modern conditions in receiving the first shock of impact and provides a cushioning and shock-absorbing medium. This can be more particularly said of men's shoes, although women's shoes with a heel up to $1\frac{1}{2}$ inches may be included, provided that the top-piece has a good surface area.

It should be understood that in good shoes there is a perfect relationship between the heel and the shoe, as the former will have been designed expressly for the shoe to which it is to be fitted. Where the shoe and heel are correctly related, weight distribution is properly balanced and the weight received in the shoe heel is passed through its centre. The higher the heel the greater is the maldistribution of weight likely to be, and in the very high heel the greater proportion of weightbearing is transferred from the heel to the ball of the foot.

When heel heights are being considered, the location of the centre of transmitted weight must be borne in mind. In standing barefoot, the centre of transmitted weight falls within the tarsal area, but as the heel is raised the weight is transferred further forward. With a heel height of over $1\frac{3}{4}$ inches the centre of transmitted weight passes from the tarsal to the metatarsal area.

Last designers have endeavoured to overcome this tendency, but there are distinct limits to what can be achieved even by the best craftsmen. As already mentioned, this problem mainly applies to women's shoes, and in giving consideration to the fitting of shoes to women the question of type of heel is a most important one. The last is designed to take a definite height of heel. This is referred to as the pitch of the last, which means that when the sole is in proper relationship to the ground, the heel of the last is elevated the correct amount to take the shoe heel. This relationship of heel height and the pitch of last is most important. It is, of course, necessary to increase the toe-spring in relationship to the increased height of the heel, and the curve of the waist will be proportionately exaggerated, and the last will be correspondingly shortened. As the heel is made higher, the pitch of the shoe is increased, and the curve of the waist correspondingly accentuated (Fig. 89). This will result in a high-heeled shoe being shorter than a low-heeled shoe of the same size.

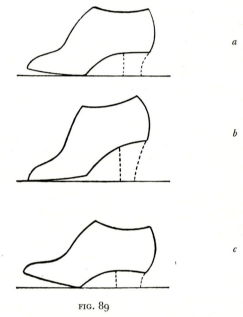

a

b

c

FIG. 89

Relationship between pitch of last and height of heel. *a*. Correct pitch of last when supported on heel of correct height. Note the space between the floor and the sole of the last which is designated the 'toe-spring'. *b*. Effect on pitch of last if too high a heel were fitted. In this instance the clearance provided by the toe-spring is eliminated by the abnormal tilt of the last. *c*. Effect on pitch of last if too low a heel were fitted, resulting in backward tilting of the last and exaggerated toe elevation.

If the last is well designed, however, and the shoe fitted with a heel made expressly for it, the toe of the foot will still have the proper clearance. This, however, is only the case where the upper of the shoe is well designed and holds the weightbearing foot firmly back, with the heel fitting snugly into the heel seat of the shoe. If the foot is reasonably flexible, a fair degree of stability can be maintained in a dress shoe with high heel if only worn for short periods, and if so worn no serious damage to the foot structures will result. If the shoe is a good fit the heel will be well seated, and the snugly-fitting rigid waist will press against the plantar surface of the instep, helping to disperse weight and preventing it all being taken by the ball of the foot. The real strain will be in endeavouring to maintain lateral stability. It is the lateral stability of the foot that is most affected by shoes of this type, even if well designed. The top-piece of a heel $2\frac{1}{2}$ inches to 3 inches high is usually very small—probably little more than 1 inch across, and often less. The waist of such shoes is also very narrow, only the central portion of the instep resting upon it, with lateral and medial portions being contracted by the upper. The tread is also quite narrow. An endeavour has been made to accommodate the foot by providing compensatory depth. Whilst the extra depth may compensate for the part of the foot that should spread transversely on weightbearing, it prevents the intrinsic muscles from functioning and undermines the stability of the anterior transverse arch, or, in other words, the base of our triangle of stability.

In the normal healthy foot, the lower and broader the heel, the greater the degree of stability. In the case of the tight tendo Achillis, the heel should be of sufficient height to allow the heel to become properly weightbearing without strain on the tendon, always remembering that the broader the bearing surface of the shoe heel the greater is the degree of stability.

In the substantial types of sports shoes and walking shoes for both men and women, support and stability can be still further increased if the following features are incorporated. Firstly, we should consider the benefit of the welted heel seat. In a shoe made with this feature, the welt is carried right round the heel. The result is that the heel counter actually sits inside the heel seat, the shoe heel being correspondingly broader. This gives perfect stability both by the fact that the heel counter does not overhang the heel, and because of the increased surface area of the heel.

Another feature that can still further support and stabilise the feet is to float or buttress the heels. This in effect means that the heel gets gradually wider towards the top-piece, giving a buttressing effect, which makes for real stability. One has only to wear shoes incorporating either or both of these features to realise the distinct improvement over other shoes.

O

SURGICAL ALTERATIONS TO SHOES

Wedges

Wedges are used to produce a tilting of some part of the floor of the shoe to alter the flow of weight distribution through the foot. The wedge should not be placed on the top of the sole or heel of the shoe but should be placed between the inner and middle soles or at the base of the heel respectively, so that the plane of the sole or heel surface itself in relation to the ground is not altered. The heel wedge should extend the whole width of the heel and should be a true wedge graduated down to a feather edge at its thinnest point. The wedge so inserted into a shoe between the heel and the heel seat will produce an angulation of the heel seat in relation to the heel.

Wedges are sometimes placed on the top of the heel or sole. The result is that there is not a uniform tilt, but an abrupt angulation at the midline which is not so effective in its results. Also, such wedges wear away very quickly and thus rapidly lose any corrective effect which they may possess, whilst repeated replacement is both costly and inconvenient. When a sole wedge is to be used, the sole should be detached from the welt or middle sole and the wedge inserted between them. In this way the proper tilt is achieved and the plane of the sole in relation to the ground remains unaltered, and as in the case of the inserted heel wedge, the wedge does not become worn and therefore retains its corrective influence whilst it remains in position.

Heel Wedge

The medial wedge is the one most frequently fitted, being used in foot strain and the milder degrees of pronated foot. Its object is to tilt the floor of the heel seat and by so doing re-align the calcaneum with the tibia. The degree of wedging is governed by actual requirements, dependent on the severity of the case and the degree of angulation of the calcaneum to the tibia. The actual thickness required can be ascertained by the insertion of experimental wedges beneath the patient's heel. This form of wedging is sometimes carried out in conjunction with the Thomas heel. The Thomas heel has already been referred to elsewhere. This is sometimes referred to as an extended heel, the extension being approximately ¾ inch (Fig. 90).

In connection with the wedging already described, the heel extension should be on the medial side. The best guide would be that the extension should be between the tuberosity of the navicular on the medial side and the anterior margin of the malleolus on the lateral side, the thickness of the wedge varying between $\frac{3}{16}$ inch and $\frac{3}{8}$ inch. The lateral heel wedge is not so frequently used, and is mainly employed for conditions usually designated weak ankles, which repeatedly turn over when walking on uneven surfaces. The lateral wedge is also used in conjunction with a lateral Thomas heel mainly for talipes varus.

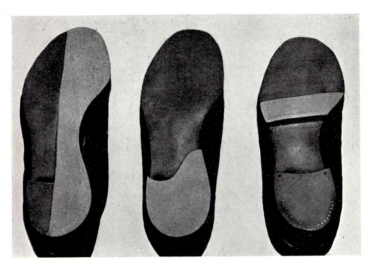

FIG. 90

(*Left to right*) Medial Thomas wedge; Thomas heel; Thomas bar.

Buttressed Heel

Heel wedging is also utilised in conjunction with buttressed heels. The buttressed heel is particularly helpful in ensuring stability, and is most beneficial when used with both medial and lateral heel wedging (Fig. 91). A combination of lateral Thomas heel with wedge and buttress is frequently used most successfully in the establishment of stability in cases of talipes varus, although in some cases the heel extension is carried forward to a greater extent, frequently filling in the whole of the waist on the lateral side. The author has almost invariably utilised a lateral buttress in conjunction with stabilising surgical insoles (Fig. 104).

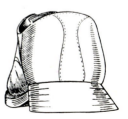

FIG. 91

Drawing of shoe, showing heel with lateral buttress.

Sole Wedges

The medial sole wedge is occasionally used in conjunction with the medial heel wedge in cases of genu varum and genu valgum, but it is often found more effective where the waist is filled in on the medial side and the wedge carried through as a continuous wedge from heel to toe, the medial Thomas wedge.

The lateral sole wedge, however, is used frequently in conjunction with the medial heel wedge in the treatment of pronated foot. The use of the lateral sole with the medial heel wedge in a treatment of this condition is to introduce the necessary corrective twist to the foot. Thus the medial heel wedge inverts the heel and the lateral sole wedge everts the forefoot and depresses the first metatarsal. The lateral wedge is also used in the treatment of varying degrees of talipes varus.

A modified form of sole wedge is the toe wedge which is placed obliquely across the toe on the medial or lateral side. The medial toe wedge is used in children to correct in-toeing, and the lateral wedge out-toeing (Fig. 92).

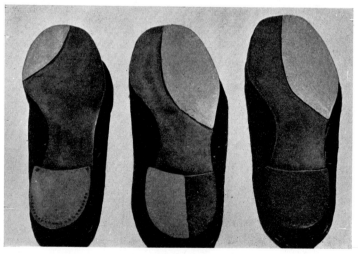

FIG. 92

(*Left to right*) Medial toe wedge; lateral sole and medial heel wedge; lateral sole wedge.

There are times when it is required to try out the effect of a wedge temporarily or it is not considered worth wedging a badly worn shoe. The same effect can be obtained by cutting an insole pattern in cortex or fleshing leather and adhering thin cork wedging to the undersurface with rubber solution. Provided there is sufficient room within the shoe this simple alternative proves quite satisfactory and it can be used also as a permanent device. It is particularly useful in school clinic work.

The fitting of all wedges should be done with the greatest possible care. Patients should be seen at frequent intervals so that the practitioner can observe the reaction to this form of treatment. Experience will show that a great variation in wedge thicknesses will be required in dealing with different cases. In many instances in the treatment of pronated foot, the heel wedge may need to be appreciably thicker than the sole wedge, or vice versa. The necessity of experimenting with wedges under the foot until the necessary corrective twist or stabilising effect appears to have been achieved cannot be too strongly stressed. The thicknesses of these wedges are then measured and wedges of corresponding type and thickness fitted to the shoe. This will avoid to a great extent a blind trial and error technique.

It is important that the patient, or in the case of children the patient's parents, should be made fully conversant with the objects which the practitioner is trying to achieve. Intelligent understanding on the part of the patient of what the practitioner is endeavouring to do will induce a more ready co-operation and a better understanding of the necessity of frequent visits often attending this form of treatment in its early stages.

TRANSVERSE AND LONGITUDINAL BARS SOLE EXTENSIONS AND PLATFORMS

Metatarsal Bar

The metatarsal bar, or Thomas bar, is probably one of the oldest and most common methods of treating defects of the anterior transverse arch. The original Thomas bar consisted of a bar of leather fitted to the sole of the shoe, and so positioned as to lie obliquely across the sole immediately posterior to the heads of the first and fifth metatarsal bones. The bar, which was about $\frac{1}{4}$ inch deep at its anterior margin and about $\frac{3}{4}$ inch wide, is kept on the same plane as the sole by building it up with a wedge piece. Thus the bar is appreciably deeper at its posterior edge. The object of the bar is to receive the first impact of weight and by acting as a lever to bridge the metatarsal heads and thus relieve the painful pressure points.

Whilst conceding the beneficial results achieved by this device in many instances, practitioners have always been conscious of its anatomical and physiological imperfections. Being a straight bar it takes the shortest route to pass between two points, viz. the first and fifth metatarsal heads. As the second, third and fourth metatarsals protrude appreciably beyond the first and fifth, the support to these areas is considerably weakened. This is particularly so in the case of the second metatarsal. Many modifications have been introduced in an endeavour to eliminate some of its defects, and so improve the device whilst retaining its principles.

The Crescent Bar

In an endeavour to follow the curve of the metatarsal heads, a bar was introduced which curved forwards. The depth and width of this bar is the same as that of the Thomas bar. This form of bar, however, obviously tends to concentrate the lever action at the most forward point of the curve (Fig. 93).

The Kidney Bar

This form of bar is strongly advocated by Brachman, who emphasises the flexibility of its application. Stating that either the broad or narrow end can be placed at the medial or lateral side, according to the pathology of the case, he also points out that either end can be wedged for the same reason (Fig. 93).

The Mayo Bar

Devised as a modification of the Thomas bar, the Mayo bar was first fitted in the clinic of the Mayo brothers. The thickness of the bar at its anterior margin is the same as the Thomas bar. It is, however, not straight, but follows the curve of the metatarsal heads. The bar is about 1 inch wide at the ends and 1½ inches at its widest point. The special feature of this form of fitment is the curve of the forward edge and the wider surface area (Fig. 93).

Anterior Heel

This form of metatarsal support is similar to the Mayo bar, but is considerably wider, extending back on to the waist of the shoe at least 1 inch further than the Mayo bar. The device is built up to maintain the surface at the same plane as the sole, to which it acts as an extension (Fig 93).

The Inserted Wedge Bar

One defect of the superimposed bar is the tendency to catch on a carpet, etc., causing the patient to stumble. In an endeavour to

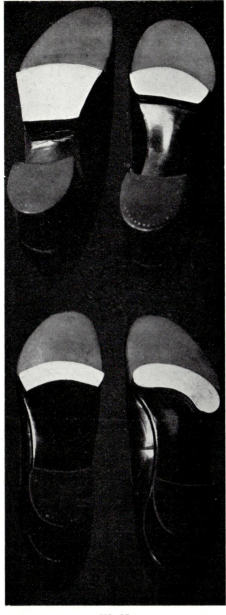

FIG. 93

(*Top left*) anterior heel. (*Top right*) Mayo bar.
(*Bottom left*) crescent bar. (*Bottom right*) kidney
bar.

overcome this difficulty and also that of rapid wear, some practitioners have inserted a piece of leather between the outer sole and the middle sole to produce the same lever action as the metatarsal bar. The shape of the thickening produced provides a distinct rocker action.

Rocker Bar for Hallux Rigidus

This form of bar, unlike the metatarsal bar, is half round in section and of the same thickness all through. It is dissimilar to the metatarsal bar in that it is placed across the metatarsal heads instead of behind them. The bar is rounded to assist in producing a rocker action. The mechanics of the device is to compensate for the lack of hinge movement in the first metatarso-phalangeal joint by a rocker action across it. Experiments have also been carried out in the form of an insertion between the outer and middle sole as a modification of this device.

Stiffening of the Uppers

It is frequently advantageous to strengthen or stiffen the uppers of a shoe, either to support weakened structures or to resist a malthrust. The old method of achieving this was to strengthen the part with leather, but it is now possible to stiffen the upper of the shoe by using cellulose cement and suitable cotton bandage or crinoline.

To obtain a satisfactory result, it is advisable first to clean the inside of the shoe, where the strengthening is to be applied, with a little of the cellulose solvent. It may be necessary to thin down the cement with solvent to make it flow freely on the brush. Apply a coat of the cement to the part to be strengthened, and then press on a strip of the fabric. Repeat the process until three or four layers have been applied. To finish the job neatly and leave a smooth surface, it is advisable to apply a final cover of soft leather, either a piece of basil split or glove kid will be suitable.

A reinforcement of this kind is most useful on the lateral side of a shoe in the case of slight talipes varus, particularly if the shoe heel is buttressed.

Stiffening of the shoe upper on the medial side to support a valgus pad will frequently be found most effective. The reinforcement is carried from the medial side of the heel down to the first metatarso-phalangeal joint. The valgus pad, which is of surgical sponge, is secured in place by using rubber solution after the stiffening has dried out. The soft covering leather is applied after the rubber pad has been secured in place.

Balloon Patch

It is frequently found necessary to dispense with the patient's normal shoe during the treatment of an acutely inflamed bunion, even when the acute stage has been safely passed. The wearing of the ordinary shoe is often not possible, particularly as dressings have to be accommodated. It is in such cases that the balloon patch will be found most useful, as in this way the additional room is provided.

An old shoe more or less discarded by the patient is useful for this purpose. An aperture is made in the shoe-upper over the joint, and a soft leather patch is solutioned in place over this. The patch is fitted in such a way as to make it bulge out like a large blister. Hence the alternative name of blister patch. The aperture covered by the bulging patch provides a large pocket, into which the joint and covering dressing can fit. At a later stage in the treatment the patch can be reduced, as the bulky dressings are now found to be no longer necessary. Patches of this type are also most effective when applied over chronic corns occurring on the lesser toes.

This work, in the opinion of the author, is a job for the shoemaker, who is skilled in his craft, and will carry it out neatly. It is not advisable for the chiropodist to encroach upon this work, which requires much training and experience, being part of the craftsman's training.

Widening the Vamp

Another surgical alteration that is often most useful is the widening of the shoe over the vamp. This is the area between the first and fifth metatarso-phalangeal joints.

In the case of a welted shoe it is usual to cut loose the welt at the side, skive the bottom margin of the upper and apply a patch with the object of providing more material with which to let out the upper. When the patch has been secured in place, the welt is stitched to the new piece of leather and the sole secured to it. Quite a considerable amount of additional room can be provided in this way.

Cut-out for Calcaneal Exostosis

A very useful method of providing accommodation for a troublesome posterior calcaneal exostosis is to cut the stitching round the top of the upper in the area of the heel. When this has been done, the upper and lining are pressed down to expose as much of the stiffener as possible. A U-shaped piece is now cut out of the back of the stiffener, large enough to accommodate the exostosis, after which the lining and upper are pulled back into the normal position and stitched. By this alteration the hard stiffener is removed from the area over the exostosis or bursa, which is now covered only by soft leather. The pocket provided can be deepened by the use of the swan-neck stretcher.

Improving the Ankle Fit

Various methods can be employed for improving the fit of the shoe round the ankle. One method is to obtain a piece of strong wash-leather, of appropriate size, and skive it thin round the margin. The leather is now folded over at the top to a depth of about $\frac{1}{2}$ inch and secured with solution. The wash-leather is now placed in the shoe with the folded portion fitting level with the top of the shoe, being secured with solution, and stitched round the top. Another method is to stitch a roll of velvet round the top of the shoe. One of the best methods, however, is again the work of the craftsman. A waxed thread is prepared with a bristle at one end and a small tight knot at the other. A hole is made in the upper, about $\frac{1}{4}$ inch down and level with the breast of the heel, and the wax thread passed through until the knot is reached. The wax thread is now laced round the top of the shoe, carrying it round the back of the heel until a position is reached level with the starting-point. The thread is now pulled very tight and the upper slightly puckered or gathered in, after which the thread is secured with another knot and the surplus cut away. The knots are now tapped flat. It is surprising how much the heel fitting can be closed in by this method. The lacing of the thread is done by making a series of holes and passing the bristle through them.

A method of improving the ankle fit of laced shoes, which is worth noting, is to pad the tongue of the shoe with felt, as this is the equivalent to thickening out the instep. A further method is to have two additional eyelet holes made, one at each side of the upper, just clear of the top eyelet holes in the shoe. This method enables the very top of the shoe to be drawn in tighter when the shoe is laced.

Stretching Shoes

It is often very helpful to be able to ease a shoe over a particular toe or across the vamp. It is also at times quite useful to be able to raise the top of the toe-box, and thus relieve pressure on the toe-nail. There are two main types of stretchers which are in common use.

The General Purpose Shoe Stretcher

This is a machine possessing two forward arms, which come together or open at the instance of a worm screw, operated by a windlass. These forward arms hold two metal fittings which are so shaped as roughly to resemble two halves of the forepart of a shoe. There are usually three pairs of these fitments which are to be used for men's, women's and children's sizes respectively. These metal shapes have a number of perforations situated on points where it is desirous to exert the greatest stretching strain, namely over the first and fifth metatarso-phalangeal joints, and situations equivalent to the dorsal aspects of the lesser toe joints, into which metal studs are fitted. Another fitment is designed to hook into the heel of the shoe, and is attached to another wheel operating a screw shaft. To stretch the shoe, the metal studs are placed in the metal shapes at the desired points. The shoe is now placed on the stretcher and the heel piece hooked in position. The wheel operating this portion is turned, drawing the hook back until it is tight in the heel, and holds the shoe on the forepart stretcher. The windlass which operates the forepart of the stretcher is now turned, separating the forward arms and causing a transverse stretching to be brought to bear on the vamp of the shoe, the greatest strain being exerted on the portion where the studs are situated.

It is not advisable to exert too much pressure on the leather at once, but to apply the stretching strain gradually, applying a few turns for a while and then applying another turn or two. It is far more satisfactory to leave the shoe on the stretcher for a few days after the final stretching pressure has been exerted, as this will ensure that the stretching is maintained.

Swan-neck Stretcher

This is a simple form of stretcher which is designed not unlike a pair of coal tongs. The two portions are 'S'-shaped and are joined by a screw. One end of the device is formed into hand-grips, whilst at the other, one portion is formed into a ring, and the other a ball. When the hand-grips are closed, the ball fits into the ring.

To use this stretcher, the ball-shaped end is placed inside the shoe at the point to be stretched. As the hand-grips are squeezed, the leather is pressed by the ball into the ring, stretching it into a bulge or blister. This machine is for very local application, and requires a great deal of exertion on the part of the operator to produce substantial permanent stretching. A good plan is to exert the necessary pressure and then tie the handles with string, so that the shoe can be left with the stretcher in it for a reasonable length of time (Fig. 94).

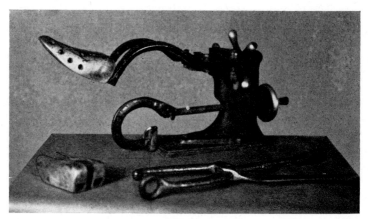

FIG. 94

Device in the background is the largest standard type of stretcher: the swan-neck type stretcher is in the foreground.

SHORTAGES

A true shortage of a limb which can be measured from the pelvis to the medial malleolus is designated a *structural shortage*. Such a shortage remains fixed both on weightbearing and at rest.

A shortage due to the contraction of muscles controlling a limb is really a pseudo-shortage. In a shortage of this kind, which is termed a *postural shortage*, the measurements from the pelvis to the medial malleolus are the same in both limbs, but measurements from the umbilicus to the medial malleolus show the variation in length if the muscle spasm is retained whilst the patient is in a recumbent position. Shortages are met with combining both structural and postural elements, but in such cases the apparent shortage on weight-bearing will be found to be greater than the shortage measured at rest. Whilst it is not possible to correct structural shortages by mechanical means, such shortages can be accommodated.

Slight shortages, say of $\frac{1}{4}$ inch or a little more, can be disregarded as they can be accommodated by the body without difficulty, irrespective of the type of shortage.

In making an accommodation appliance for a structural shortage, such as a cork elevation for the shoe, Brachman suggests that for a shortage of less than $1\frac{1}{2}$ inches it is only necessary to elevate the heel and mid-tarsal area, the additional weight thrust being taken by the ball of the foot, but if the fixed shortage is greater than this it is necessary to extend the elevation beneath the ball of the foot to achieve an even distribution of weightbearing through the foot.

Cork Elevations

Cork elevations of a moderate nature, 1–2 inches, can be fitted to stock shoes if a collar is fitted to the shoe uppers.

In the more severe shortages, however, it is usually necessary to fit a cork sole and heel extension (Fig. 95).

In many cases requiring surgical boots with cork elevations it is not always possible to achieve a perfect distribution of weightbearing, and as a result painful pressure areas result. In such cases painful calluses and even trophic ulcers result from the friction and pressure.

It is in such cases that the authors' technique of grafting the plastic surgical insoles to the cork elevations has proved so beneficial, particularly if the cushioned-surfaced type of insole is used (Figs 96-98). The success of this form of appliance

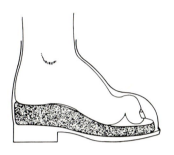
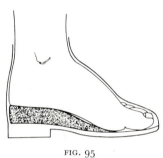

FIG. 95

Examples of cork elevations.

is due to the absolute accuracy with which the surface of the appliance fits the plantar surface of the foot. In this way complete diffusion of pressure is ensured, and the comfort of the appliance is achieved by its cushioned surface. These combined elevation appliances have proved consistently successful in many cases of severe talipes equinus.

In recent years, since the great increase in bespoke footwear as a result of the advent of a national health service, an economic method of producing these shoes has become generally adopted.

Large quantities of second-hand shoe lasts are purchased. A person termed a fitter takes the required measurements of the patient's feet and also drafts of the feet. Upon these drawings are marked any special features to be considered. These measurements with the appropriate information are passed on from the shoe-fitter to the last-fitter, who is usually a shoe-maker. He selects from the lasts available a pair nearest to the measurements supplied. He then makes such alterations as are required to achieve the measurements referred to. This is done by building up the lasts with leather.

There is one great weakness in this method. The last shape and build-up of the last is done by a person who has not seen the patient's foot. He has, therefore, nothing to assist him, other than position marks on the plantar drawings (drafts), in achieving the correct measurement and form at any point. Thus, although he may achieve the correct joint measurement in the circumference of the joint, the displacement of the volume can often be quite inaccurate. Although all the measurements may be correctly complied with in the shoe, it may not fit the foot as the displacement of the volume at various points may be wrong, allowing too much room at one point and too little at another.

Therefore, in this method of bespoke shoe-making, the end results are frequently very disappointing in appearance with a very high percentage of misfits. This, however, appears to be the most prevalent method of surgical shoe-making used today. This problem could be reduced considerably if full-foot casts were taken of the patient's feet so that the last-fitter could use them as models and thus build up the contours of his lasts to correspond with those on the casts. This, of course, would add considerably to the expense of making the shoes, quite apart from the fact that one would have to ensure that the fitter was skilled in the making of such casts.

In the United States, where the problem of making bespoke shoes down to a price does not arise so acutely, bespoke footwear of a high standard can still be obtained. Even there the number of skilled shoe-makers available is still very limited, though the craftsmen of Europe have been drawn to the United States over the last twenty-five years.

The American podiatrists have, however, attempted in various ingenious ways to produce orthopædic footwear not only to fit their patients' feet correctly, but also to embody therapeutic qualities with the co-operation of the shoe manufacturers.

No doubt there are several makers of this type of footwear who employ variations in the processing techniques. In most instances, casts of the feet are the basis of these shoes. Material is added to the ends of the toes to provide the toe clearance and the shoe is made round these casts. They are usually without a heel, being the platform type; the toe shape follows the natural toe line embodied in the casts.

The resultant shoes look very large and certainly have no claim to beauty, and whilst they are often very successful functionally, they have never really fully established themselves with the public generally on account of their appearance. Certain principles are, of course, embodied in these shoes, namely the accurate plantar contours of the foot with the toe crest.

Another form of shoes which are produced by a different technique have also proved functionally successful and in the case of the ladies' shoes they have a somewhat more presentable appearance. These custom-mould shoes are made already in a range of sizes and fittings and contain removable cork inlays. The inlays have a lip all round the margin.

The first procedure is to select a pair of these shoes of the correct size and fitting. The inlays are then removed and marked with chalk or a pencil at the points where allowance is to be made for bony prominences in the foot, such as bunions, enlarged sesamoids, tailor's bunion, depressed metatarsal heads or hammer toes, in fact any pressure points.

Pockets are now ground out at these points using a rotary file. A compound which is supplied with the shoe is mixed and trowelled onto the inlay where it is held by the lipped edge. The foot is then placed on this inlay within the shoe to produce a dynamic inlay (Chapter 10).

The full detailed instructions for fitting shoes of this type and preparing the inlays are supplied by the manufacturers. It is my intention to give only a general survey of the principles on which this system works. A sandal is also available using this technique. In this case, however, the inlay is the sole of the sandal and is not detachable. Like the previously mentioned type, this technique is used very successfully with patients who are amenable to this type of footwear.

There is one thing to be said for both these techniques. They are based upon very sound principles and with the co-operation of the patient they can be very successful.

CHARLESWORTH LASTS AND SHOES

The Charlesworth last is a new and unique solution to the problem of ensuring a correct fit in a bespoke or surgical shoe.

The design and method of preparation of these lasts are the result of many years of investigation, research and experiment which have resulted in a scientific method of last-making whereby a perfect replica of the foot is produced and converted into a modern shoe last.

The hazardous and uncertain procedure of taking measurements and tracings often results in an indifferent fit, and bespoke and surgical shoes so measured are often devoid of character and poor in appearance. With the Charlesworth last such uncertainty of fit is replaced by certainty, and the appearance is improved to such an extent that surgical shoes are almost indistinguishable from normal ones. These qualities arise from the accuracy with which the last can be produced and the manner in which displacements and deformities of the foot can be accommodated and concealed. To achieve this the last incorporates the most advanced orthopædic features ensuring comfort, correction and stability. The design also permits such combinations as a moccasin appliance or splint boot to be accommodated within the Charlesworth shoe in addition to any built-in corrections which may be necessary.

The basis upon which this last is built is a cast of the foot, the impression for which needs to be taken in a special way. This entails the use of the casting machine described earlier (Chapter 2). The machine is set up to give the heel height and waist curve required for the finished shoe. A plaster of paris bandage is used to take the actual impression and before the plaster sets the foot is placed on the machine. The foot is then moulded into the corrected position required under sufficient pressure to ensure that the heel is weightbearing and that there is adequate joint spread, i.e. that the downward pressure applied to the foot spreads the forefoot out almost but not quite as much as it will spread in walking. Correct heel-spring and waist curve are automatically incorporated by the machine, together with adequate toe rise for the heel height chosen. On removal of the plaster the foot is measured with the tape at the ball, instep and heel and the overall length is measured under weightbearing with the size stick. The impression shell should be filled with a hard-setting plaster. Just before setting a short piece of metal pipe should be inserted in the leg part, flush with the top of the plaster to make a socket for mounting the last on the shoe-makers' stake. Any of the hard- or stone-setting plasters are suitable for filling but a very useful and tough plaster can be made by mixing equal parts of superfine dental plaster and Polyfilla. When the plaster has hardened and the cast has been removed from the plaster of paris bandage, it is set aside to dry out. When dry the measurements of the foot are checked against it. The cast must now be corrected so that its measurements are very slightly full on those of the foot. This is necessary to ensure that the internal volume of the finished shoe accords with the shape of the foot and is achieved by adding fresh plaster or scraping plaster away as necessary. One must now decide upon the overall length of the last. To a certain extent the style of shoe desired by the patient affects this. The toe can be styled broad or long to meet the patient's needs or wishes but the normal allowance of two to two and a half sizes ($\frac{2}{3}$–$\frac{5}{6}$ inch) over the foot size is given. This can be varied according to the style of the shoe or the degree of flexibility or rigidity of the foot. This extra length is added by building a toe extension onto the cast in hard plaster or plaster/Polyfilla mixture. This extension is shaped to suit the needs of the patient and the style of the shoe desired. Sufficient of the mixture is applied to the sole and sole borders of the cast to permit of shaping the cast to true last contours. The back part of the cast is now reduced below the malleoli to ensure a close fit of the shoe round the ankle. The foot measurements are again checked against the cast to ensure accuracy.

The cast has now been converted into a last upon which the footwear can be built. Since it will be necessary to break the plaster last out of the footwear when made, it is advisable to make a copy of the last by a hot moulding gelatine process in case subsequent pairs are needed.

The last now incorporates correction for position as well as heel height and toe rise. This latter needs to be increased if stiff-soled footwear is envisaged in order to compensate for the lack of flexibility in walking. If, however, flexible-soled shoes are to be made, the toe rise need not be increased provided that the metatarsal-phalangeal joints of the patient are also flexible. If these joints are greatly restricted in range then a stiff-soled shoe with the greater toe rise will be more comfortable.

If it is considered that the patient will require a built-in insole with flanges for stabilisation or a soft insole with cushion pads for comfort, this should now be prepared and made ready to go onto the last so that the shoe can be built around both last and insole. In this way adequate room can be provided for the insole and any modifications needed to accommodate it either to the last or the shoe can be made.

In all essential respects the last is a normal basis for making footwear by standard methods, yet it provides for the making of a shoe which will be a perfect fit having eliminated the sources of error which normally occur.

From a simple bespoke shoe for a foot with but minor defects to one for the accommodation and stabilisation of a foot with gross deformity, every contingency can be met with by this method. Only Charlesworth shoes are made on lasts prepared and developed in this way and this system has finally evolved a method for the successful resolution of the most difficult fitting problems. It does, however, require the co-operation of a skilled and willing surgical

P

boot- and shoe-maker who understands the special problems involved and who holds a licence to make footwear by this method under the patents governing it. The name and address of such a company is to be found in the directory of suppliers provided at the end of this book.

15

A Selection of Interesting Cases

THIS chapter was compiled with the object of providing a small selection of cases (each different in character) in which the author has employed in his treatment, in some form or other, one of the appliances described in this book.

The assessment in each case has been carefully recorded to enable the reader to follow the author's reasoning in arriving at his conclusion, as to the type of appliances to be used, in approaching the solution of each individual problem.

It is also desired to convey by this chapter some idea of the scope and immense possibilities of this field work.

Male Aged 58 Years

History. This patient with a history of anterior poliomyelitis as a child was referred to me by an orthopædic surgeon. As a result of this disease and subsequent wasting of the limbs, the condition terminated in a typical talipes equinus with considerable shortening.

Examination. The examination revealed painful callosities around the margin of the heel, ball of the foot and the dorsal aspect of the great toe. Careful checking of the patient's surgical boot and cork elevation showed that the latter was a very indifferent fit in relation to the contour of the plantar aspect of the foot. There was a distinct space between the surface of the cork and the long arch. On weight-bearing, excessive weight was borne by the heel and the ball of the foot. The foot tended to be precipitated forward into the toe of the shoe, resulting in a back pressure on the great toe, producing a severe hallux flexus. Dorsal pressure on the toe caused the formation of a chronic corn and underlying bursa. The back pressure on the ends of the toes aggravated the subluxation of the metatarso-phalangeal joints, and was a contributory factor to the formation of the painful callosities on the ball of the foot.

Assessment. My conclusion, as the result of this investigation, was that an indifferently fitting cork elevation whilst giving the correct degree of lift had failed to provide stability for the foot. Instead of fitting truly to the contour of the plantar surface, thus holding it securely and diffusing pressure, it merely provided a sloping platform down which the foot was precipitated. This forward progress being arrested by the end of the shoe resulted in the symptoms previously

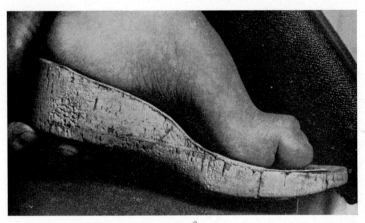

FIG. 96

Talipes equinus. Poorly fitted cork elevation showing space between the instep and the cork.

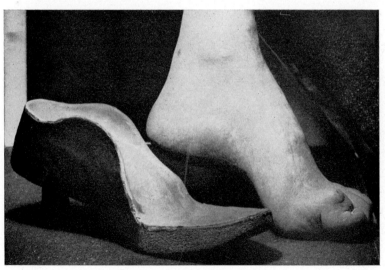

FIG. 97

The appliance and the patient's foot.

Note. The double-flanged surgical insole is grafted onto the cork elevation.

described. It was therefore decided to make a double-flange surgical insole on a cast of the foot; the metatarsal area being provided with a cushioned surface. This cupped heel, double-flange appliance was grafted onto the cork elevation, and resulted in the patient being provided with a fitment in his surgical boot, which embraced accurately the whole plantar surface of his foot. The cupped heel and the medial and lateral flanges contributed a bracing effect, whilst the cushioned anterior surface supported the metatarsal region. The absolute accuracy of the fit of this appliance resulted in complete diffusion of pressure and secured and stabilised the foot in the proper

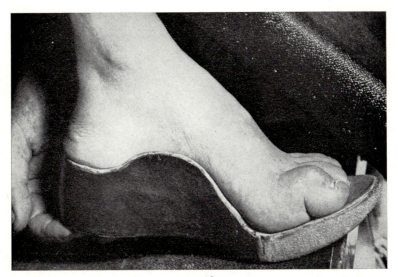

FIG. 98

The foot in position on the appliance.

position in relation to the boot. Previous to the fitting of this appliance, the patient had suffered considerable pain and was receiving chiropodial treatment fortnightly, but had experienced very little relief.

In the first twelve months following the fitting of the appliance, treatment had only been necessary on four occasions. During these visits, it was noted that the patient had experienced only a little discomfort rather than that of actual pain, and the callosity was considerably reduced. During the second year a replacement appliance was fitted, and further chiropodial treatment has not been found necessary (Figs 96, 97, 98).

Male Aged 30 Years

History. This patient who had a history of anterior poliomyelitis as a child was referred to me by a foot hospital.

Examination. There appeared to be a long history of severe metatarsal pain for which regular chiropodial treatment had given a measure of relief. The patient had been referred because it was felt that possibly relief of a more positive and permanent character could be achieved by the fitting of appropriate appliances. The left foot showed a condition of severe pronation, with subluxation of the metatarso-phalangeal joints of the lesser toes and valgus deviation of the great toe. It was obvious that the condition of the left

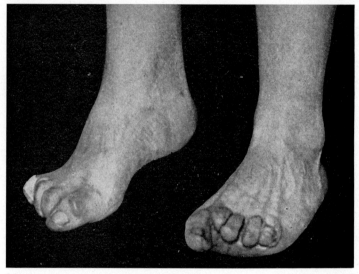

FIG. 99

Clinical picture of feet showing talipes equino varus (*right*) and pes planus and retracted toes (*left*).

foot was due to taking the greater degree of active and passive strain. As the result of the disease previously referred to, the right foot showed a condition of talipes equino varus, with clawing of the toes and hallux flexus, which had in turn produced painful corns.

Assessment. In dealing with this case, two distinct types of appliances were necessary. In the case of the left foot, a corrective insole for pronated foot was fitted, with a sponge surface anterior metatarsal support. For the right foot, it was decided to make a cushioned surface insole with a lateral buttress and the necessary anterior

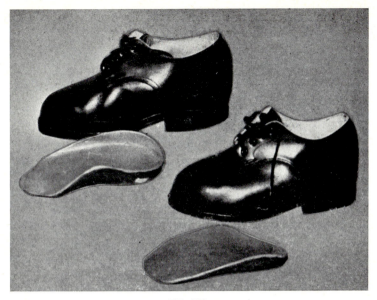

FIG. 100

Surgical shoes and appliances. Note elevation incorporated in the appliance for the right foot.

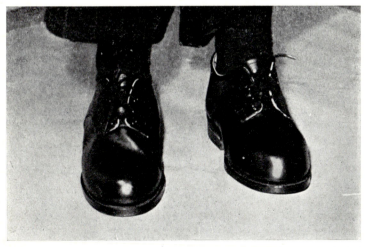

FIG. 101

Patient wearing appliances and surgical shoes.

metatarsal support. It also incorporated a cork elevation appropriate to the shortening of the limb. It is obvious that appliances of this nature require surgical shoes to accommodate them. The necessary shoes were made, and in the case of the right foot the heel was designed with a lateral buttress. Once again the combination of appliances and surgical shoes proved highly successful, the patient saying he had never walked with so much comfort before (Figs 99, 100, 101).

Male Aged 55 Years

History. This patient was referred by his doctor on the advice of an orthopædic surgeon. He was a very severe case of kyphosis.

Examination. The examination of the patient's feet showed a severe condition of talipes varus, more marked in the left foot. The strain on the lateral malleoli resulted in large ganglionic swellings. The cuboid bones were very large and prominent, being subjected to severe pressure and friction, resulting in the formation of large and painful callosities. In the case of the left foot, the lateral thrust was

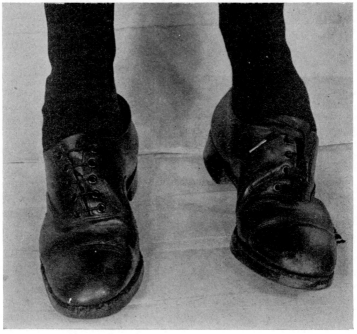

FIG. 102

Talipes varus. Note the supination and inversion of the left foot. The burst welt can be clearly seen on the lateral side.

so great as to burst the welt away from the shoe. The patient was quite unable to gain any degree of stability, and locomotion was erratic and staggering.

The treatment of this patient was rendered more difficult owing to his hypersensitivity to his condition; as an example of this, he was adamant in his objection to the wearing of surgical boots.

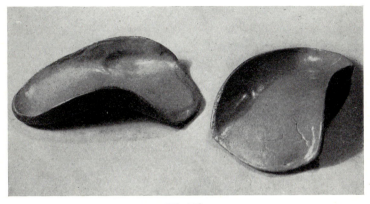

FIG. 103

Stabilising appliances, showing depression to accommodate the cuboid bones.

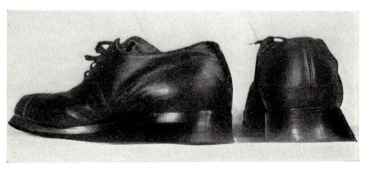

FIG. 104

Surgical alterations to shoes, showing lateral extension and buttress.

Assessment. The object in this case was to achieve the best degree of stability possible by countering the lateral thrust and relieving as much as possible the strain on the lateral malleoli. Casts of the feet were made and surgical insoles designed, each with a strong lateral buttress. Special accommodation and soft padding had to be provided for the cuboid bones. The stabilising effect of the appliance was further improved by a deep cupping of the heel. A pair of new shoes, of the type previously worn by the patient, were fitted with lateral buttress heels. The heels were extended on the lateral side to fill in the whole of the waist of the shoes, and the buttressing was designed with a very marked flare.

The combination of the insoles and the alteration to the shoes produced a marked improvement in the stability of the patient. A diffusion of pressure was achieved by the accurate fit of the appliances. This was particularly applicable to the cuboids, where the perfect cushioning provided complete protection. The strong lateral flange received the initial thrust, and assisted in relieving the strain on the malleoli.

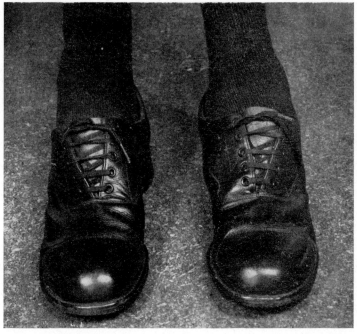

FIG. 105

The same patient with appliances and shoes fitted with surgical alterations.

In this case the beneficial effect of the appliances could not be achieved without the important shoe modifications. The lateral buttressing and extending of the heels succeeded in stabilising the appliances in the shoes, which produced a combination resulting in a marked corrective effect on the feet. When wearing the shoes and the appliances the patient was able to stand and walk without the assistance of sticks (Figs 102, 103, 104, 105).

Female Aged 65 Years

History. This patient who was suffering from arthritic flat foot was referred to me by an orthopædic surgeon.

Examination. The patient was complaining of severe pain when walking. The condition had reached the distressing stage when locomotion had become a misery to the patient, and showed every prospect of reducing the patient's mobility to the absolute minimum. A Keller's operation had been performed on the first metatarso-phalangeal joint of the right foot for hallux rigidus. The middle three

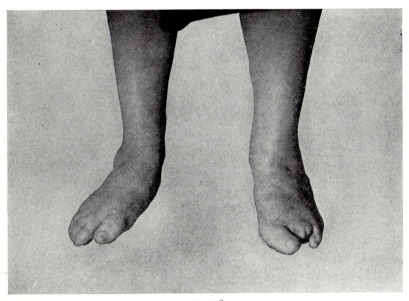

FIG. 106

Arthritic flat foot. Note amputation of middle three toes, left foot. Keller's operation, right foot.

toes of the left foot had been amputated because of gross deformity; there was also a severe valgus deformity of the great toe. With regard to the long arch, whilst there was some flattening of the feet, the condition was mainly one of pronation. Arthritic changes had resulted in an absence of movement in the tarsal and sub-taloid joints.

Assessment. In cases of this nature the pain arises as the result of stress upon the joints seriously affected by advanced arthritic changes. In such cases it has been found that a rigid appliance as distinct from a semi-rigid arch support is advisable. It was decided in this case to make rest appliances of a rigid type, with a cushioned surface. Inside flanges were provided which were continued down in the form of buttress walls to receive the medial thrust. Again, the principle of diffusion of pressure was introduced, the insoles being

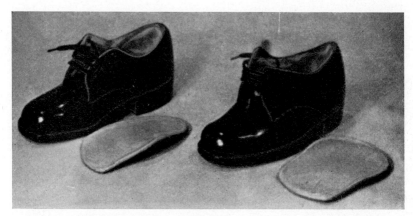

FIG. 107

Shoes and appliances. Note the broad-waisted shoes and rigid rest appliances.

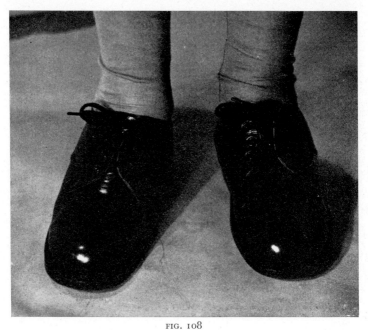

FIG. 108

The patient was successfully stabilised by combination of the shoes and appliances.

made on casts of the patient's feet; the pressure was evenly distributed over the supporting surfaces by the perfect relationship of the contours of the superior surface of the appliances and the plantar surface of the patient's feet. The squaring off of the medial flange assisted in stabilising the appliances in the shoes, and countering the tendency to tilt over under pressure of the feet when weightbearing. The layer of surgical sponge on the surface of the appliances provided an initial cushioning and shock-absorbing effect. In cases of severe pronation of this nature, the appliances are essentially broad and cannot be satisfactorily fitted in ordinary stock shoes. Therefore, in this case, surgical shoes were made with the broad waists necessary to accommodate and stabilise the appliances properly. The shoes were also fitted with floated heels to assist still further in establishing the complete stability of the feet. This combination of insoles and surgical shoes proved to be a distinct success. All the points aimed at in the assessment were achieved, i.e. elimination of pain, relief from strain of the joints and complete stability of the feet (Figs 106, 107, 108).

Female Aged 26 Years (Lobster Claw Feet)

History. This congenital deformity was inherited from her father and passed on to her male child. The patient attended Salford Royal Hospital, where she was fitted with bespoke shoes to accommodate the unusually shaped feet. The case was referred to me at Hope Hospital with a view to stabilising the feet.

Examination. Examination of the feet revealed that in the case of the left foot there was a marked degree of pronation due to an elevation of the first metatarsal. There was a valgus displacement and elevation of the great toe. In the case of the right foot, the elevation of the first metatarsal was very marked, but a hyperflexion of the great toe compensated for this and stabilised the medial arch. Excessive friction and pressure, however, beneath the inter-phalangeal joint of the great toe had resulted in a painful callosity. A severe lateral thrust on the fifth metatarso-phalangeal joint and along the plantar surface of the fifth toe had also resulted in painful callous formation.

Assessment. On the basis of the examination of the case I decided to provide a rest appliance for the left foot which would support the foot against the tendency to pronate. A build-up of cork on the appliance beneath the first metatarsal was incorporated to take up the space between the elevated first metatarsal and the floor of the shoe. A firm inner flange also assisted in the stabilisation of the foot, and in combination with the cork build-up prevented pronation. The appliances which were made upon a cast of the plantar surface of the foot was cushioned with surgical rubber sponge. By this combination of the medial build-up and diffusion of pressure the foot was stabilised. In the case of the right foot, two factors had to be considered; one was the painful pressure area on the inter-phalangeal joint of the great toe due to hallux flexus, and the extreme friction and pressure beneath the fifth metatarso-phalangeal joint due to the severe lateral thrust. In this case the appliance was made with the object of complete diffusion of pressure. Cork build-up was

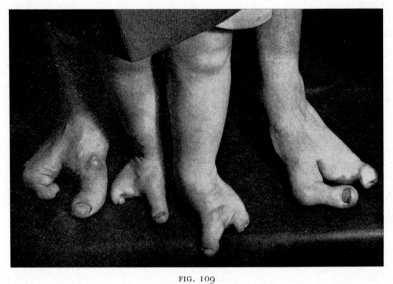

FIG. 109

Lobster claw feet. Showing identical duplication of the mother's feet in the male child.

carried along the medial side to the base of the inter-phalangeal joint to take the weight off this painful area. The appliance was flanged and buttressed on the lateral side to receive the thrust and relieve the strain on the fifth metatarso-phalangeal joint. A latex and sponge rubber shield encased in wash-leather—on the toe glove principle—was made to fit on the fifth toe and metatarso-phalangeal joint. The padding was situated along the plantar surface to provide a cushioning effect. The appliances fitted in the bespoke shoes perfectly, and when wearing the appliances in the shoes the patient was not only perfectly comfortable but an extremely satisfactory psychological effect was achieved of added confidence in herself. She not only felt stable and walked with greater confidence but the posture and gait were distinctly improved. It is hoped by the experience gained in treating the mother that satisfactory treatment of the child can be undertaken.

It would be unwise, however, to assume a successful conclusion of this case on the basis of the initial success (Figs 109, 110, 111, 112, 113).

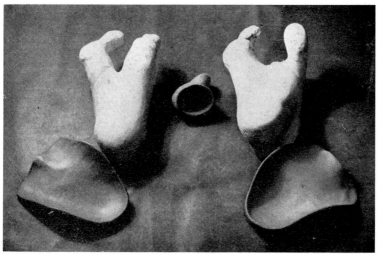

FIG. 110

Casts and appliances. Note the contours of the superior surface of the appliances.

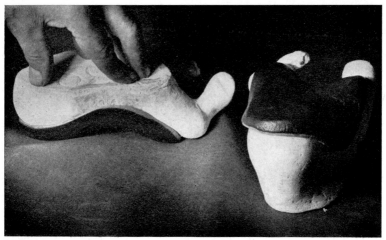

FIG. 111

Note the perfect fit of the appliances to the casts.

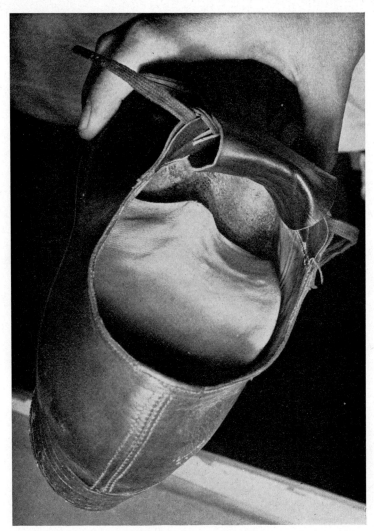

FIG. 112

Appliance fitted in the left shoe.

Woman Aged 45 Years

History. This patient who was suffering from a long-standing condition of arthritis was referred to me by a chiropodist.

Examination. The patient complained of extreme pain on the ball of the foot and the ends of the toes, with intermittent pains in the feet generally. Gross deformity of the toes had occurred, resulting

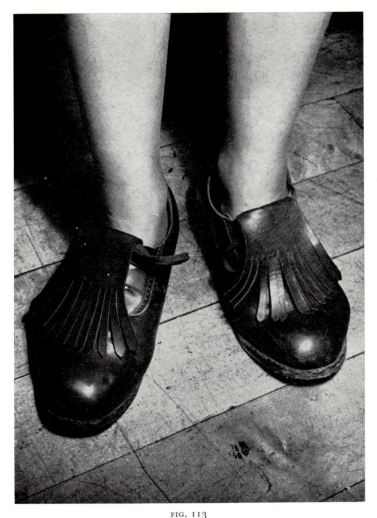

FIG. 113

Patient wearing the surgical shoes and appliances. Note the fringed tongue
style to hide the peculiar shape of the feet.

in the formation of painful distal corns. The second toe on the left
foot and the second and third on the right had been amputated.
There was a severe hallux valgus deformity of the left foot and some
degree of hallux flexus on the right. A subluxation and arthritic
changes in the metatarso-phalangeal joints had resulted in painful
callosities. The patient had been receiving chiropodial treatment

Q

which had proved the only means of obtaining any measure of relief, but had reached the stage when the repeated application of pads and plaster had induced a deleterious action on the skin in the form of a severe plaster dermatitis over the metatarsal area.

Assessment. It was decided that a straightforward moccasin appliance was the best means of dealing with this condition. A combined valgus pad and metatarsal support in surgical sponge was built onto the appliance. The metatarsal pad was extended as a bevel over the metatarso-phalangeal joints. A sponge rubber overlay was applied over the whole plantar area, and extending over the ends of the toes. These simple and uncomplicated moccasins proved completely effective. No further symptoms were experienced by the patient. After five months' wear a review of the case was carried out. The result was astonishing; not only was there a complete absence of any dermatitis, but the callosities had also disappeared. The dry keratotic condition of the skin previously noted had given place to the soft and silky tissue of a young and healthy foot. The second pair of appliances have been recently fitted, and the patient is quite happy, experiencing no symptoms (Figs 114, 115, 116).

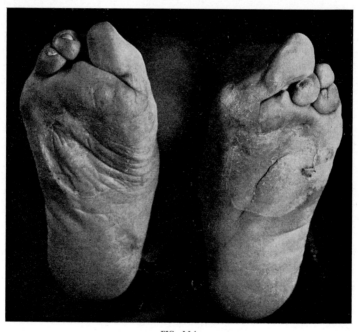

FIG. 114
Deformity of lesser toes and plaster dermatitis on the plantar surface of the feet can clearly be seen.

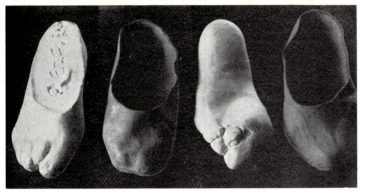

FIG. 115

Plaster casts of the feet and the moccasin appliances.

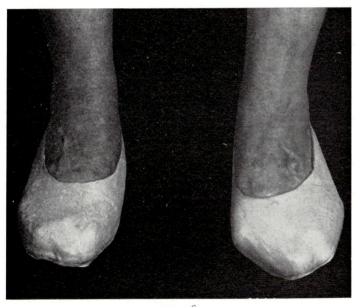

FIG. 116

Patient wearing the moccasin appliances.

Girl Aged 14 Years

History. This patient who was a post-operative accident case was referred to me by an orthopædic surgeon.

Examination. The patient complained of extreme pain over the suture areas and certain pressure points on the anterior plantar

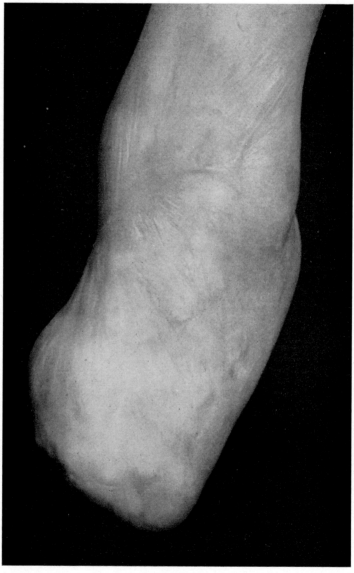

FIG. 117

Post-operative accident case. Girl aged 14 years. Suture areas can be plainly seen.

margin of the foot. Owing to the absence of sufficient subcutaneous tissue, there was insufficient natural cushioning of bony prominences. As the result of the severity of the accident, there was considerable scar tissue in the region of the malleolus. There was a deep cleft situated in the centre of the plantar surface of the foot anteriorly, resulting in pressure being thrown onto the anterior margin. The general circulation in the foot was extremely poor.

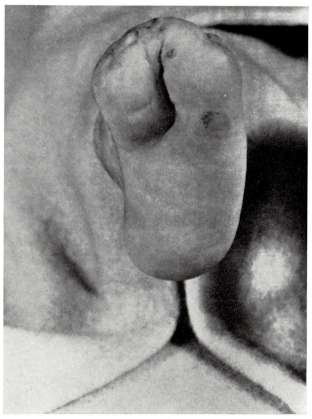

FIG. 118

Same case showing deep cleft on plantar area.

Assessment. A moccasin appliance was decided upon to provide a soft and resilient support and a measure of insulation. On the plantar surface, padding was introduced into the cleft to ensure pressure diffusion; valgus padding to give support to the medial arch was also introduced. In making the first appliance, plantar

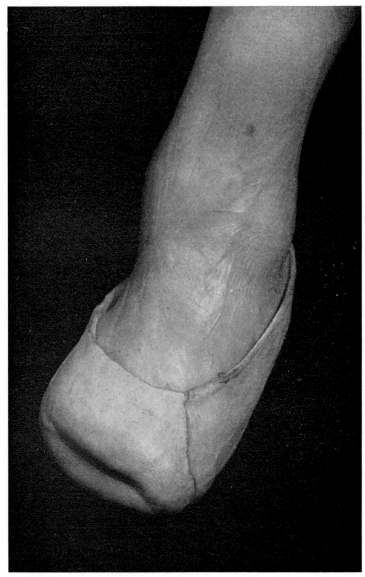

FIG. 119
Moccasin appliance fitted on the foot.

padding of latex foam was carried forward over the anterior margin onto the dorsal surface, and further padding over the anterior margin was provided with the object of building up a very soft and resilient buffer. The appliance had a lining of fine chamois leather. This appliance was, however, not successful; so exceptionally sensitive were the suture areas that even the fine, soft chamois leather and soft, resilient sponge could not be tolerated. After giving considerable thought to the problem, a new moccasin was made in which anterior padding was provided by a buffer with an aperture. The buffer was so designed as to receive the pressure on the upper and lower margin, allowing the suture areas to rest in space. Plantar padding was still further improved by supporting the two anterior pressure areas.

The appliance proved perfectly successful, the foot was reasonably stabilised and there was a complete absence of symptoms. It is six years since the first successful appliance was fitted. Three replacements of a similar type have been provided.

There is some improvement in the circulation, the scarred appearance of the tissues around the malleolus has greatly diminished; whereas on the first appearance the ankle was puckered and shrunken, it has now filled out to normal proportions, and in thin silk stockings compares favourably with that of the other (Figs 117, 118, 119).

Male Aged 78 Years

History. This patient was referred from an old people's institution by the consultant chiropodist. The case was a gross talipes equinus deformity with a slight varus deviation.

Examination. The patient complained of painful callosities on the ball of the foot. The callosity was very considerable and complicated by a corn with a deep-seated nucleus situated over the head of the fifth metatarsal.

The extreme angulation of the foot resulted in the subluxation of the metatarso-phalangeal joints, causing a direct thrust on the metatarsal heads.

The patient was wearing an old felt boot, many sizes too big. The severe pain considerably restricted the patient's mobility.

Assessment. It was obvious that the object of any appliance in this case would be to provide a satisfactory means whereby the thrust on the heads of the metatarsals could be received and cushioned.

A cast of the foot was taken and considerable experiment was carried out. The resultant appliance was a corset-like device which embraced the tarsus. The plantar portion was carried forward to the base of the toes, and heavily padded with surgical sponge and appropriately moulded with suitable depressions. The margin of the anterior plantar portion was formed into a cushioned roll, which, fitting as it did into the crook of the toes, provided a supporting prop. The appliance was lined with chamois leather, which was also carried forward over the anterior roll. The tarsal portion was divided down the front and fitted with eyelet holes and a lace. When

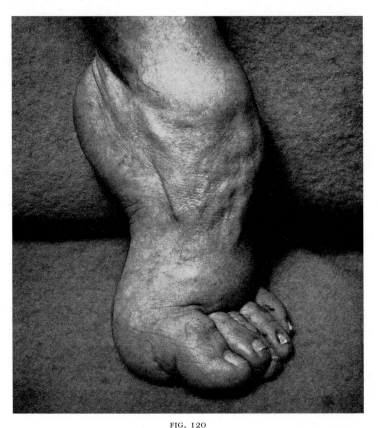

FIG. 120

Extreme talipes equinus with slight varus deviation. Patient aged 78.

laced in position, the appliance fitted securely and snugly to the foot, the toes protruding from an aperture formed between the anterior roll and the dorsal portion.

A suitable boot was designed to accommodate the foot and the appliance. The result was most gratifying; a complete absence of the symptoms was reported by the patient, who is now completely mobile, and has been free from pain over a considerable period of time. This result has been maintained, and there is every indication that the success of this solution of the problem is permanent (Figs 120, 121, 122).

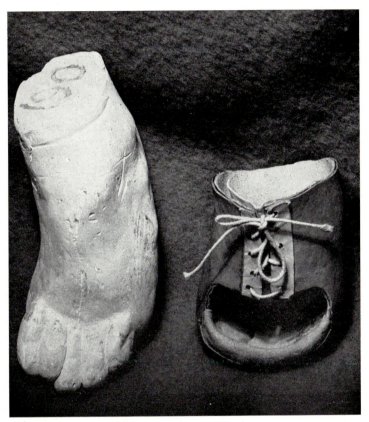

FIG. 121

Cast and finished appliance.

Girl Aged 14 Years

History. This was a case of spina bifida, referred from the orthopædic department of a general hospital. Ulceration had resulted in erosion of all toes, except the fourth on the right foot.

Examination. At the time the patient was examined there was a perforating ulcer beneath the first metatarsal head, with the sinus radiating posteriorly. The object in referring the case was to produce an appliance which would cushion and protect the affected area,

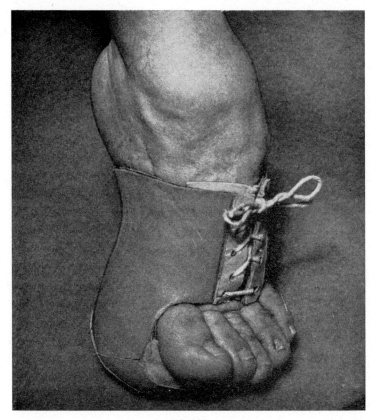

FIG. 122

The appliance fitted on the patient's foot.

and thus assist healing. There appeared to be no breaking down of the tissue elsewhere.

Assessment. In treating this condition a moccasin appliance was decided upon as being the best means of providing protective padding which could not be dislodged or displaced when the patient was walking. It was also felt that this type of appliance was easily removed and replaced during treatments of the ulceration. The device was designed with a valgus pad extending to the metatarsus and a soft cushioning portion with a marked depression over the opening of the sinus. The surgical sponge was so shaped and formed as to receive the weight on the valgus pad, and the outer portion of the metatarsal extension. The overriding pressure on the area of the ulcer was taken by the additional soft cushioning, and the depression over the sinus provided protection from any pressure.

This appliance proved successful in providing the necessary protection of the affected area, preventing irritation and the breaking
down of the tissues at other weightbearing points. It also considerably assisted the frequent change of dressings. In several
similar cases, ulceration of long standing has promptly responded
to the fitting of these appliances by rapid healing where previously
the tissues had invariably broken down and ulcerated when the foot

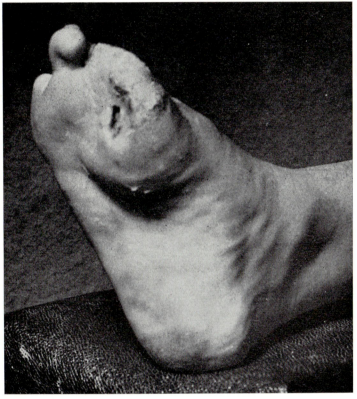

FIG. 123

Perforating ulcer with sinus radiating back over the metatarsus.

had become weightbearing. The continued wearing of these appliances in such cases has maintained healing.

It is felt that one of the most important functions of an appliance
in cases of this nature is to provide protection and prevent the
breaking down of the tissues as a result of friction and pressure
(Figs 123, 124, 125).

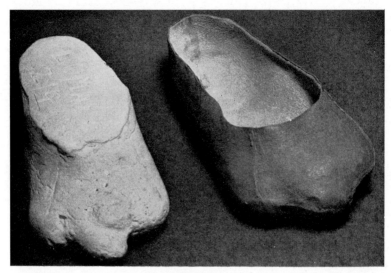

FIG. 124
Cast and moccasin.

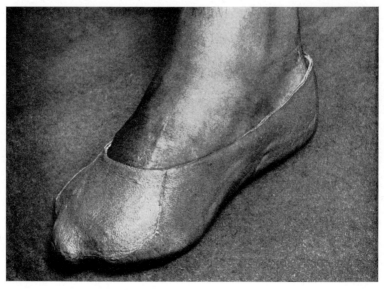

FIG. 125
Patient wearing the moccasin appliance.

Female Aged 17½ Years

History. This case of congenital absence of toes was referred to me by another chiropodist.

Examination. On examination it was noted that in the case of the left foot the tarsus was normal, in the right foot the cuneiforms had not properly developed. As a consequence, the anterior portion of the right tarsus was narrower than that of the left. The medial arch was very distinct, with a deep cleft extending along the tarsus, causing an acute concavity. The prominence of the heads of the first and fifth metatarsals resulted in painful plantar callosities, which

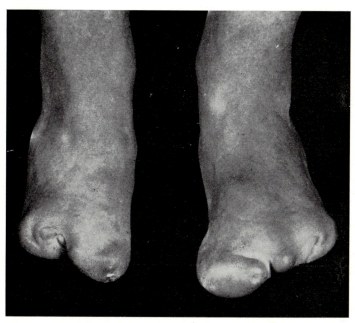

FIG. 126
Congenital absence of toes. Girl aged 17½ years.

extended onto the anterior margin. The flexibility present in the normal foot was absent, causing the patient to be unstable on weightbearing. It is interesting to note that in the case of the left hand of this patient there was a congenital absence of the fingers. Not only had the patient a considerable degree of discomfort and a measure of instability, the footwear also constituted a serious problem. Another aspect of this case was the psychological effect of these deformities on the patient, who had become markedly conscious of being an oddity.

Assessment. In approaching this case I felt that I had three problems to solve; firstly, to provide relief from pain, secondly, to establish stability, and thirdly, to provide an appearance of normality. Casts were taken and experiments were carried out in designing a suitable moccasin appliance. The moccasin was so designed as to provide support for the medial arch and to relieve pressure from the two

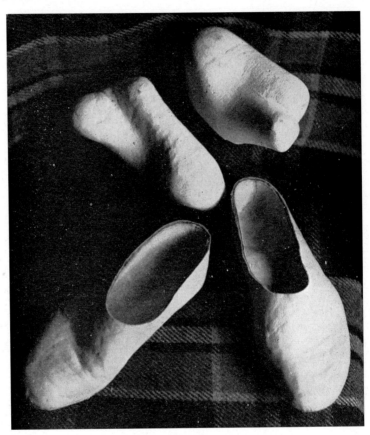

FIG. 127

Casts and finished moccasins.

anterior pressure points. This was achieved by fitting sponge rubber valgus pads with lateral extension, passing forward into the deep groove in the anterior portion; in fact the whole of this depression was completely filled in. A sole piece of thin sponge was now fitted over the whole plantar surface and carried forward over the anterior margin of the appliance.

The next step was to build up and shape the false forefoot; before doing this, however, I felt it advisable to fill in the hollow on the lateral side of the tarsus on the right foot so that its contour matched the left. The reason for this was to ensure that the finished appliances were the same size and properly matched, and so would fit correctly in a normal pair of shoes.

A false forefoot was shaped and built up from segments of surgical sponge. When worn with stockings, these appliances gave the appearance of perfectly normal feet. Stability was achieved, firstly, by the sponge valgus support and, secondly, by the false forefoot.

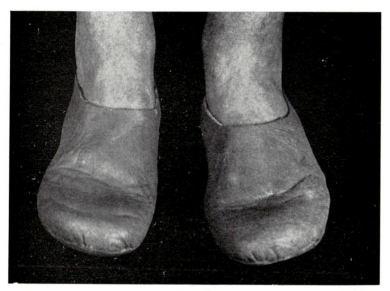

FIG. 128

The patient wearing the appliances.

The false forefoot played an important part in establishing stability by reconstructing the equivalent of the hinge action of the metatarso-phalangeal joints, and by the degree of the resistance offered when the foot was bent in walking, inducing a similar action as that which occurs when the toes press against the sole of the shoe, an important stabilising factor often overlooked.

These appliances were exceptionally effective, all symptoms disappeared and stability was established. The stockinged foot presented a normal appearance and the patient was able to fit and wear ordinary shoes. These not only looked normal in wear but retained their shape in use, owing to the resilient forward extension filling and padding out the front of the shoe. The patient has now been wearing these moccasins for a considerable time; an endeavour has been made to improve her last pair further by making a liberal number of perforations all over the uppers of the appliances to assist aeration, and reports on this innovation are awaited (Figs 126, 127, 128, 129).

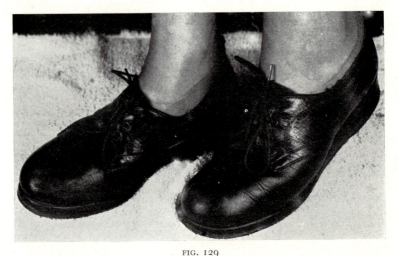

FIG. 129
The patient wearing normal shoes with the moccasin appliances.

Girl Aged 5

History. This patient was referred to me from another hospital. This girl had only the fifth metatarsal and toe on each foot, the cuneiforms were undeveloped, but the other tarsal bones were normal. There was complete absence of toes and metatarsus, with the exception of the fifth metatarsal and fifth toe. It is interesting to note that the child's father had similar deformities. The patient's hands are similarly malformed, only a portion of the hand and the little finger being present.

Examination. The fifth metatarsals and toes were set at an abnormally oblique angle to the rest of the foot. Absence of the metatarsus and most of the tarsus on both feet resulted in the feet falling over onto the navicular in weightbearing, which is equivalent to pronation in the normal foot. In the case of the left foot there appeared to be an abnormal thrust on the fifth metatarso-phalangeal joint, the condition being characterised by the presence of a callosity. On the right foot there were signs of abnormal pressure and friction on the anterior aspect. It would appear that slight bony prominences were inducing the formation of bursæ and callosities. It should be noted that whilst the plantar surface of the left foot was more or less concave, that of the right foot was convex.

Assessment. It was decided to make a pair of moccasin appliances with a sleeve for the fifth toe. As the fifth toe of the right foot tended to elevate, it was decided that the sleeve should be braced on the plantar surface with the object of pulling the toe down. An operation to fix the toes at a more convenient angle was refused by the parent. It was hoped—if the parent had consented—to set the fifth toe into proper alignment with the rest of the foot. A false forefoot of latex foam could have been built on, to which the sleeve of the fifth toe

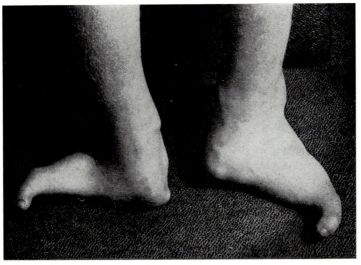

FIG. 130

Congenital absence of toes, showing the feet weightbearing. Note the angle of the fifth toe.

could have been anchored, and the whole of the appliance formed into the shape of a natural foot. As the parent was not agreeable to radical treatment, it was decided to carry out this principle as far as possible, taking into account the angles of the fifth toe. The moccasins were made with a firm texture of surgical sponge built up beneath the naviculars as a wedge, to provide a level surface area for the feet and stabilise them in the correct position. A sleeve for the fifth toe was included in both moccasins. The sleeves were fixed to a false forefoot of surgical sponge in such a way as to exert traction in an endeavour to bring the toes into more normal alignment.

R

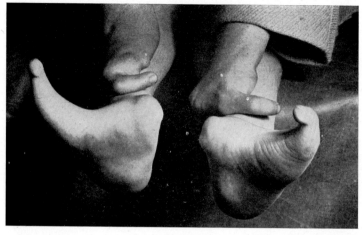

FIG. 131

Congenital deformity. It will be seen that the hands have a similar defect to the feet. Note the pressure areas beneath the central metatarsal area, right foot, and the fifth M.P. area, left foot.

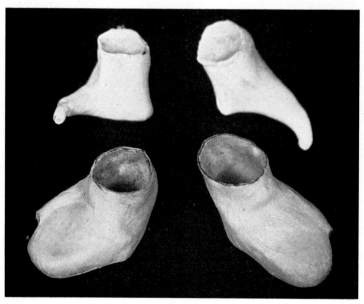

FIG. 132

Casts and finished appliances.

Surgical shoes were made to accommodate the child's feet wearing the appliances. The child is at present wearing the shoes and appliances. Whilst not actually painful, traction of the fifth toe right foot is giving a little trouble, but it is hoped that this will be overcome in due course (Figs 130, 131, 132, 133).

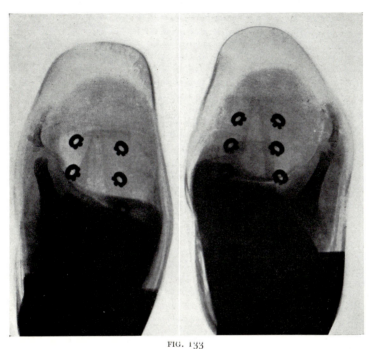

FIG. 133

Radiograph showing position of toes in the shoes. Outline of the appliances can be clearly seen.

Girl of 11 Years with Paresis of Lower Limbs due to Spina Bifida with Meningocele

This patient was referred by the orthopædic consultant of a special school. She was unable to stand or walk unaided as her legs crumpled up under her. Her feet and legs were anæsthetic.

An endeavour had been made to enable her to walk by the making of surgical boots with steel splints up the legs and thigh-length calipers. This method had proved very disappointing. The limbs sagged against the calipers and the ankles impinged upon the splints with the result that ulceration occurred in a short time. The effort to walk using these thigh-length calipers also proved very distressing. The result of this effort was that a short and distressing period of trial was, on each occasion, followed by a long period confined to bed healing severe ulceration. The poverty of circulation made healing a long and difficult process with the result that further attempts at walking were abandoned. It was as a result of my success with moccasins in several cases of spina bifida that I was invited to see this particular patient. I did not feel that the use of calipers in this case, even with a protective moccasin-type boot, would provide the answer. The child found the effort required too great; and had become apathetic and completely disinterested in efforts made to get her walking.

In spite of this a start had to be made and a pair of moccasin-type appliances were made for her but two difficulties were encountered. One was that the toes became folded under the foot as the moccasin was put on and the other was that the feet still sagged inward on weightbearing so that the inner ankles still came into contact with the calipers. It became obvious that a bootee type of appliance would be needed with the sole stiffened and the toes propped up. This was an improvement but the toes still curled under as the appliance was put on and the feet still sagged inward in spite of foam rubber medial arch padding.

I therefore decided to take full lower limb casts and build boots upon them in which the lining was soft chamois leather. Over this I moulded soft latex foam and applied splintage down either side. This splintage was composed of layers of cellulose acetate-soaked scrim and bandage and, since this will not adhere to latex foam, an intermediate layer of scrap leather pieces was applied. The appliances were then completed in the manner of a moccasin and removed from the cast by cutting down the front. The area over the dorsum of the toes was removed, the cut edge down the front was bound with leather strip and eyeleted to take a lace and the sole was stiffened with an extra layer of leather. It was in this manner that the splint boot was born which has since been modified so successfully to deal with post-polio and other suitable cases.

When the splint boots were finished I had a pair of surgical boots made to accommodate them. I prescribed heels that were flared and extended on the medial sides to provide a firm buttress that would resist the inrolling stresses of the feet and help keep them firm and level. It was arranged also for the child to be supplied with elbow crutches for use with the splint boots and surgical footwear.

By some mischance these were all sent to the child's school for fitting and not to my clinic. As I was rather apprehensive as to the

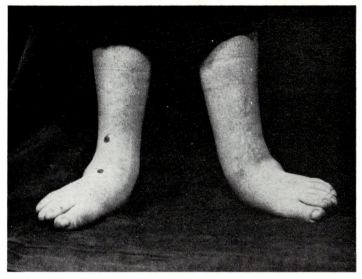

FIG. 134

The patient is being supported on her feet; even so the feet inroll badly.

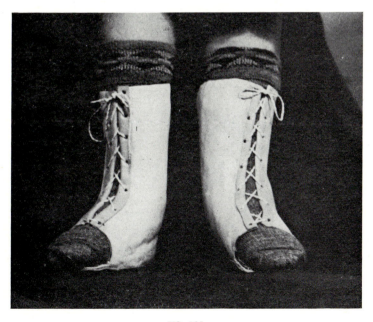

FIG. 135

The splint boots on the patient's feet. She is standing unsupported. Compare foot positions with Fig. 134.

manner in which the child might take to the appliances, I wished
to fit them myself but my fears were groundless for, when brought
to my clinic by ambulance, she walked in beaming, wearing the
boots and appliances quite unaided, except for her elbow crutches.

It is now six years since the first splint boots were fitted but the
girl has been maintained on her feet ever since. Ulceration has
occurred on occasions but has been of far lesser severity and at long
intervals. The girl has also been able to go home to her family for

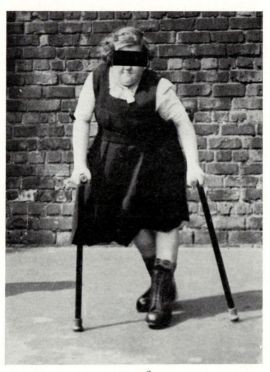

FIG. 136

The patient walking with elbow crutches. The surgical boots were specially
made to take the splint boots inside.

regular periods of holiday and at most weekends. Above all she has
been able to participate in the normal activities around her and her
mentality has shown a remarkable improvement.

It is interesting to note that, whereas strong thigh-length calipers
were not able to provide support, the lightweight splint boots were
completely successful.

In the clinical photographs you will see the child, who is supported by two adults, with her legs dangling and the feet toppling into pronation (Fig. 134). You will also see her standing in the splint boots which are capable of supporting her fully weightbearing with no assistance even without the surgical boots (Fig. 135). She is also seen walking alone with the aid only of her elbow crutches (Fig. 136). The photograph of the left appliance shows how careful control of the foot during the process of impression taking enabled an appliance to be built which has slight pitch into inversion to counter the strong eversion of the foot under weightbearing (Fig. 137).

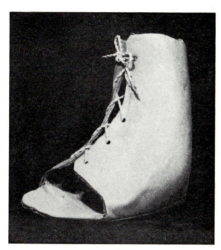

FIG. 137

Splint boot for the left foot. Note the inversion twist which was applied to the foot in casting. This counters the eversion twist which occurs on weightbearing.

Severe Pronation in a Child of 5

This boy of 5 was sent by an orthopædic surgeon on account of severe pronation. On examination he was found to have long thin feet and on standing he rolled into extreme valgus foot (Figs 138 and 139). He showed the worst pronated feet ever seen in this hospital.

The extreme length and narrowness of the feet made him unstable both in standing and walking. He soon wrecked his shoes as they were unable to withstand the tremendous inrolling of the feet. The boy made some subconscious attempt to overcome this by plantar flexing his great toe and some degree of early hallux flexus was present together with enlargement of bone ends at metatarsal-phalangeal and metatarsal-cuneiform levels.

The forefoot was not as greatly abducted as one would expect to find with so much pronation but the sustentaculum tali were both thrust into very great prominence, indicating great heel eversion and sub-talar looseness. In fact all the joints of the foot were hyper-mobile. His shoes were long enough but it was impossible for him to obtain sufficient length without their being too wide.

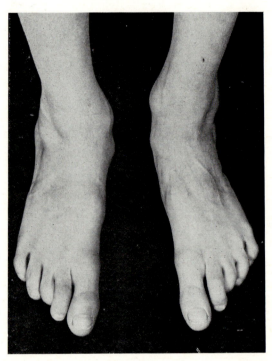

FIG. 138
Pronation on long thin feet.

It was apparent that this boy would need a pair of stabilising insoles which would invert his heels and prevent his first metatarsal from rising under weightbearing. An impression was therefore taken in putty (Fig. 140) with the heel inverted, the forefoot everted and the first metatarsal head pushed well down into the putty.

The appliance was made by stretching a dampened blocking leather onto the cast and backing this with the latex leather dust, wood flour and cork granule mixture. It was shaped, when dry, to include a good outer heel flange and long inner flange well up into the arch (Figs 141 and 142). By this means the heel eversion was controlled and the inrolling of the midfoot reduced. The foot was, in fact, screwed up by the appliance into the corrected position in which it was cast.

Standing and walking are now greatly improved, fatigue of foot and leg muscles is reduced and walking ability is greatly improved.

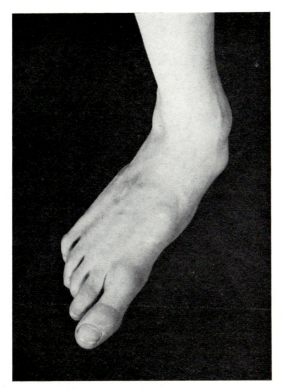

FIG. 139
Severe pronation of right foot.

So far he has had six pairs of appliances made in five years and will require further pairs as he grows. It is hoped that, by the age of 18, his feet will become naturally more stable and he might be able to dispense with the appliances altogether. Alternatively he might require a lighter form with less correction. It will, however, be necessary to keep him on this type of corrective appliance at least until he has stopped growing.

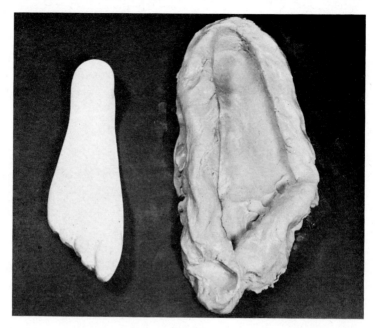

FIG. 140

The putty impression and the plaster cast. The long thin nature of the foot is
now readily apparent.

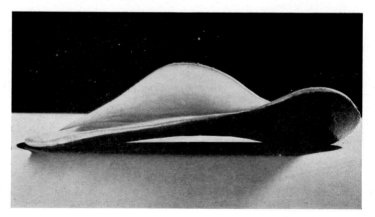

FIG. 141

Lateral view of the left insole.

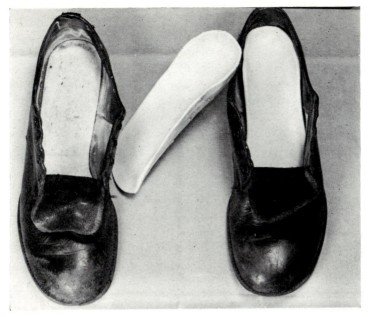

FIG. 142

The insole and shoes.

Girl Aged 2½ Years with Congenital Absences

This girl was sent by the consultant orthopædic surgeon, for a prosthetic appliance which would assist in stabilising the foot. The mother was most anxious that the girl should be able to wear normal-looking shoes.

The diagnosis was that of congenital absence of the fourth and fifth metatarsals and toes of the left foot.

To begin with moccasin appliances were made which were filled in to make up for the absences and which stabilised the foot by preventing it from rolling over laterally. She has been fitted with these for fourteen years quite satisfactorily. New ones were made to fresh plaster casts every three to six months according to the rate of growth (Fig. 143).

At the age of 16 it was decided to transfer her to surgical inlays (Fig. 144), which were capable of retaining the stabilisation without being so bulky or so occlusive. These too are replaced to fresh casts according to growth and are proving satisfactory.

It is obvious with a foot like this, that some compensatory device will always be needed if the foot is to be stabilised. With such an inlay the outlook is reasonably good; without it she would become very unstable and have difficulty in walking. At every change in shoe size and often too whenever she changes the style of her foot-wear, a new inlay has to be made as, apart from its main function of stabilising the foot in making good the absences, it fills in the space between foot and shoe and prevents the upper from collapsing and creasing. From the young lady's point of view this is probably its greatest asset. The shoe size is controlled of course by the size needed by the other foot. The inlay makes it possible to fit the affected foot with a shoe of the same size and type so permitting the purchase of pairs of shoes from stock.

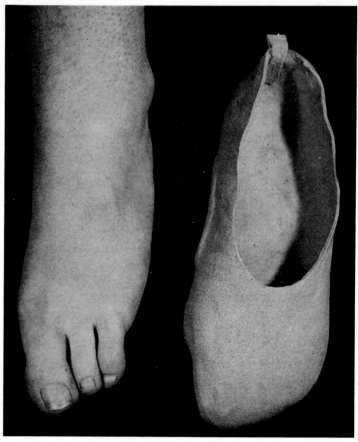

FIG. 143

Patient's foot. Note the absences. One of the first type of appliances used; a moccasin is shown on the right.

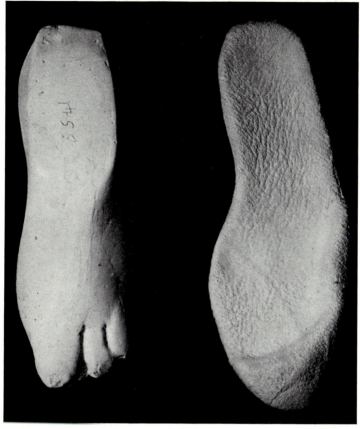

FIG. 144

A later cast of the foot and the type of insole subsequently used. This insole is covered with chamois leather. Later ones were surfaced with natural surgical basil.

Female 64 Years

This lady was referred from the orthopædic clinic on account of arthritis and deformity. The lesser toes had been amputated, as being severely hammered and painful they made shoe-fitting impossible. In addition the foot was pronated and unstable. The great toe, lacking the resistance of the lesser toes, was moving increasingly into valgus. This applied particularly to the terminal phalanx (Fig. 145).

It was decided to make her a moccasin with a toe-block for the lesser toes and a firm, closed-cell rubber arch pad. The plantar area required a soft, open-cell sponge rubber surface all through, with the addition of a soft sponge metatarsal pad shaped and fitted to

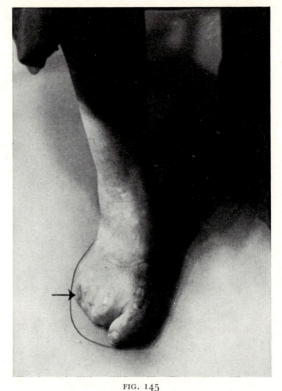

FIG. 145

The foot with toes amputated.
The arrow indicates the painful area on the fifth metatarsal head.
The curved line indicates the area to be filled in to make
dummy toes.

relieve pressure on painful and calloused metatarsal heads. The
fifth metatarsal head required special protection as it was very
painful (note arrow in Figs 145 and 146).

Specially made surgical shoes were needed to encompass both foot
and moccasin. She was quite stable in these and comfortable too,
once the moccasin was holed out over the painful fifth metatarsal
head (Fig. 146).

This appliance lasts her about twelve months and, at the time of
the first remake, she asked for a higher back to be made. A deeper
cast was taken and a high back made to the moccasin. Subsequently
the surgical shoes were also made deeper to accommodate it. This
combination of deeper appliance and deeper shoes keeps her
comfortable and stable (Fig. 147).

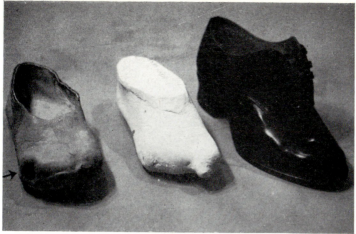

FIG. 146

The appliance, the cast and the surgical shoe.
The arrow indicates the hole over the painful fifth metatarsal head. The
thickness of soft padding around it can be observed.

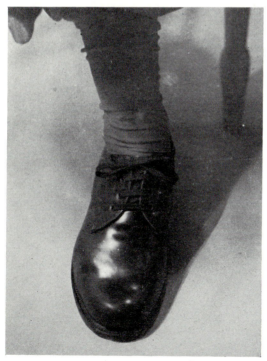

FIG. 147

The foot and moccasin within the shoe. The patient is
weightbearing.

Boy Aged 7 Years

This boy was referred by the orthopædic surgeon to see what could be done to stabilise him on an insole following surgery for a congenital lobster claw deformity (Figs 148 and 149).

A putty impression was taken and a plaster cast prepared. This was backed with thin leather on which was spread some of the leather dust, cork and wood flour mixture bonded with latex. The affected foot was considerably shorter than the sound opposite foot. A paper pattern was therefore prepared the same size as the sound foot and a leather insole was made to act as a base upon which to mount the insole for the affected foot. By this means the insole could be made

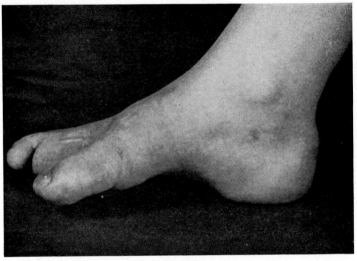

FIG. 148
Cleft foot after surgical intervention.

the same size as the sound foot with external measurements. It would then be possible for the patient to be fitted with a normal pair of shoes.

When the prepared insole was dry and hard it was removed from the cast. The edges were trimmed and the outside scoured smooth on the grinder. The leather insole base, made to the size of the opposite foot, was then adhered to its under-surface. A toe-block of the same mixture was then modelled onto the forepart to make good the lack of toes and to prevent the toe-cap of the shoe from collapsing in use. When dry this toe-block was ground smooth and covered with thin leather (Fig. 150).

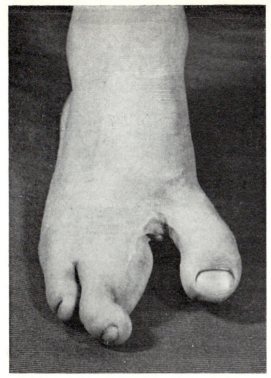

FIG. 149

Cleft foot, showing extent of cleft and isolation of the
first metatarsal and great toe.

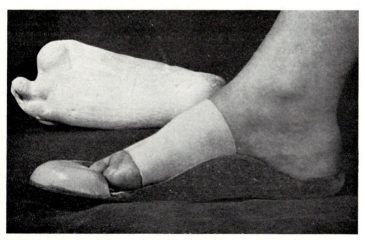

FIG. 150

The finished insole and the foot with metatarsal band. The plaster cast on
which the insole was made can be seen in the background.

S

Since much of this boy's instability was due to the isolation of the first metatarsal from the rest of the forefoot by a deep cleft an elastic metatarsal band was made to fit around the forefoot. This is worn with the insole but is quite separate from it. The combination of insole and metatarsal band is quite comfortable and by this means maximum stability is obtained (Fig. 150).

This combination of appliances has required changing about every six months as he grows. He has had six appliances between the ages of 7 and 10 and, in spite of a setback due to a fracture of the femur on the affected side at the age of 9, he is comfortable and active. Being able to wear normal shoes, his disability is not noticeable and he is not embarrassed by it (Fig. 151).

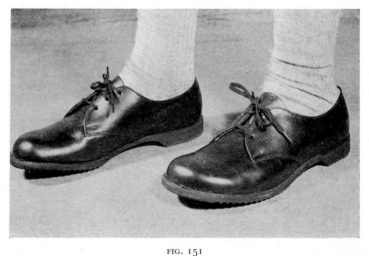

FIG. 151

The patient wearing the insole and metatarsal band standing in normal boys' shoes.

16

The Chiropodial Orthopædic Unit

THE HOSPITAL UNIT

SINCE a chiropodial orthopædic unit should form part of the hospital orthopædic service, it would be profitable to consider how such a unit can be organised and how it should function as part of that service.

It is not practicable for such a unit to be established at other than large hospitals, though it may be advisable to establish a department at one hospital to provide a service for a group, patients being referred to the chiropodial orthopædist in charge from the orthopædic departments of the various hospitals. Experience has shown that the value of such a service soon becomes apparent, and the demands upon it overwhelming.

The equipment and the administration of the department can best be outlined by describing the layout and organisation of the unit established at Hope Hospital, Salford, which is the first of its kind.

It was developed in progressive stages by Dr Charlesworth and commenced as a small processing laboratory in addition to the usual chiropody clinic. As the work grew this was found to be too small and it was necessary to design a new department in which both chiropody and chiropodial orthopædics could be carried out. The general plan is shown in Fig. 152.

The new unit is self-contained. A common waiting room serves both the chiropody clinic and the appliance section. A chiropody clinic equal in size to the previous one provides the routine chiropody treatment. A casting room designed expressly for our particular type of work is situated between the consultant's room and the processing laboratory.

It would be advantageous to describe the principal features of each room with the object of giving the reader a clear picture of the general organisation and administration of the unit.

Waiting Room

This is a small room designed to accommodate about fourteen patients. A large waiting room is not necessary, as the appointment system operates. A door leads from the waiting room to the chiropody clinic, and a sliding window between the waiting room and the consultant's office permits the receptionist to prepare case sheets and check appointments.

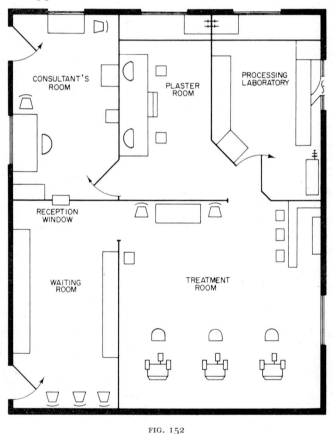

FIG. 152

Plan of chiropodial orthopædic unit.

Chiropody Clinic

The clinic is equipped with the latest form of clinical furnishings, including three treatment chairs, instrument tables, foot lamps, nail drill, etc. It is in this clinic that the orthodox chiropody treatments are carried out and the foot appliances fitted.

The chiropody clinic is also used by the orthopædic surgeon when examining patients with a view to prescribing surgical footwear. A short passage opens from this room into the plaster room.

Plaster Room

A special feature of the plaster room is a platform, equal in height to the chiropodist's stool. Upon this platform are placed the chairs for the patient. This arrangement obviates the practitioner stooping to floor level when taking plaster casts. He can sit in a comfortable position on the stool and place the patient's foot on the tray, which is at a convenient level. A casting bench and sink are situated along the end of the room which is lighted by a large window (Fig. 153).

Processing Laboratory

A door opening into a passage from the chiropody clinic to the plaster room gives entrance to the processing laboratory, which, like the plaster room, is lighted by a large window stretching almost across the whole width of the room. The laboratory is equipped with a large table designed as a cutting-out table for leather and sheet rubber. At one end of the table is situated the thermostatically controlled oven. This is useful for speeding up the curing process and drying out the leather and casts. A shoemaker's finishing machine has been installed which provides all the necessary tools for grinding, scouring and polishing the appliances (Fig. 154). A special feature of the laboratory is a processing chamber which was designed by the author and keeps the noxious vapours and fumes from being inhaled by the chiropodist or technician. Such substances as petroleum æther, cellulose cement, strong ammonia, etc., are used in the making of various types of appliances.

The chamber has a sloping top fitted with windows of Perspex. The front of the chamber is fitted with canvas sleeves and elastic wrist-bands. At one end an aperture, covered with metal gauze, provides the air intake, whilst at the other end a funnel terminates in an extractor fan which draws the air with the noxious vapours from the chamber.

The various processes are carried out by passing the hands through the wrist-bands into the chamber which contains all the necessary processing materials. The work is observed through the roof of the chamber, which is fitted with windows. This device has proved a great success. Previous to the chamber being fitted, the room was always heavy with fumes, causing headaches, because an extractor fan fitted in the window was not successful in carrying off the fumes.

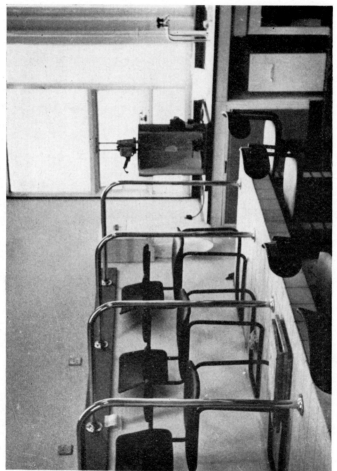

FIG. 153

Plaster room with impression taking platform and plaster mixing machine which is modified from an electric drill with a step-down gear and variable resistance in series. Access to platform by steps moved into position opposite each casting chair.

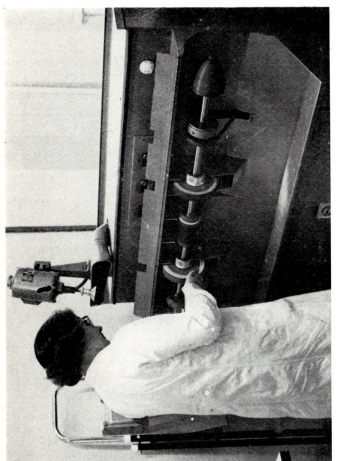

FIG. 154

Shoe repairer's finishing machine modified for foot appliance work with scratcher brush (out of view at left hand end of shaft), 1¼ inch flat, 4 inch sole and 1¼ inch curved scouring wheels. An electrically heated shaping and burnishing cone is on the right hand end of the shaft. This machine incorporates its own extraction fan. Extraction orifices are below each scouring wheel. The top guard is shown lifted to give a better view of the wheels. The Naumkeag mounted on top of the machine is useful for small pad shaping.

With the new chamber, the air in the room is fresh and quite free from noxious vapours of any kind. The processing laboratory is also fitted with benches, sink and shelves, etc.

Consultant's Office

The office, which has a separate entrance from the outside of the building, can also be entered from the casting room. The office is used for consultation between the chiropodist and the orthopædic consultant, and for personal interviews with the patient when privacy is required. The case sheets are filed in this office, and it is used by the appointments officer when the clinics are in progress. A phone communicates with the exchange and all departments of the hospital.

Record System

Patients for chiropody treatment must be referred either from their own doctor or from a department of the hospital, or another hospital or clinic. A case sheet, containing the full particulars of the patient and the history of the case, is contained in a stiff folder, which is filed in the usual way. Correspondence from the patient's doctor, hospitals, etc., is also placed in the folder for reference. Every visit of the patient is recorded on the case sheet, with the date and treatment given, and any remarks of the chiropodist giving treatment.

The cases referred for appliances have a special card, containing brief history of the case and full prescription for the appliances, which is filed in the processing laboratory and referred to when the appliances are being made. All modification to the appliances are duly recorded on this card; also observation as to fit, comfort, etc.

In cases of special interest, photographs are taken with the object of providing visual record of progress. The records are invaluable for reference when undertaking treatment for cases of similar nature.

Children's appliances are replaced every four to six months, according to age. In the case of adults the patients are recalled at appropriate intervals for examination and, if found necessary, repair, alteration or replacement of appliances is carried out. If new appliances are required, fresh impressions are taken every time. It is felt that if the appliances have had any degree of success, the feet will have altered to some extent and, in consequence, accuracy in fit requires new casts.

It should be mentioned that each patient is supplied with an appointment card, upon which is entered by the appointments clerk the date and time of the next visit.

DESIGN OF A PRIVATE PRACTICE CHIROPODIAL ORTHOPÆDIC UNIT

The development of a chiropodial orthopædic unit in private practice has made it necessary to give some thought to the design of rooms and the selection of equipment for this purpose.

It is a great advantage not to have to introduce plaster of paris and messy materials into the surgery. Dental wax sheets for bunion impressions and alginate impression compound for lesser toes make useful alternatives. It is also possible to introduce plantar impression trays of putty into the surgery prepared and powdered ready for use. All these materials permit impression taking under clean conditions and the impressions so made can be filled with plaster of paris outside the surgery.

The greatest difficulty in controlling any mess is likely to be encountered where a deep full foot cast is needed. Either the chairside area must be covered up with rubber or polythene sheeting or the casting must be done elsewhere. The simplest and possibly the cleanest method of taking a full foot cast entails the use of plaster of paris bandages but even so plaster drips are likely to be a nuisance. The exercise of great care in use and in arranging the surgery beforehand will keep these to the minimum. The ideal arrangement whereby one has a small spare room or surgery for all impression and plaster work is rarely obtainable, but it is of the greatest possible convenience whenever much of this work has to be done.

Demands on space are usually very great but whereas the plaster room is a convenience, a processing room is a necessity. It is sometimes possible to use one room as a combined plaster and processing room but it must be remembered that patients have to be introduced into this room so some means is needed of partitioning or curtaining off the processing space even if only as a temporary measure while patients are there. I do not like them to be faced with a whole workshop array of casts, machines and all the paraphernalia which go with this work. If patients are not to be brought into such a combination room, a processing room can be situated either in a cellar, upper room or even in a shed, and here impressions can be filled with plaster, the casts can be trimmed and the appliances processed well away from the main surgery.

It is possible to use all the methods described in this book in a private practice but most practitioners will prefer to master one or two methods of making each type of appliance to simplify the ordering and storage of materials and to be able to organise longer production runs. The processing together of a batch of the same sort of appliances lends itself to considerable economy in both time and materials and has much to commend it. Working under private practice conditions I have found the latex dip method, using pre-vulcanised latex, for dorsal digital and hallux valgus appliances to be both economical and remunerative. For toe props I now prefer the silicone rubber method. Neither of these methods entails the purchase and use of fine and expensive chamois leathers but I have met some practitioners who tell me that they prefer non-casting methods of making these pads with open-cell sponge rubber, chamois covers and strip rubber loops, as being more convenient. These are usually the people who like to make their digital appliances at the chairside with the patient present all the time. Other people will take impressions and make the appliances out of sight after surgery hours. It is all a matter of preference and of accommodation being available outside the surgery, but consideration must be given to all these points before a decision can be made as to the planning of appliance rooms.

Plantar appliances mostly involve more work and only the simplest of the non-casting techniques can be carried out entirely in the surgery. When impressions are needed for plantar work the making-up of the appliances usually requires the use of some sort of grinding machinery.

If anything more than the simpler chairside types of appliances are intended to be made, a special making-up room is essential. This room should, for single-handed working, be not less than 6 feet by 8 (Fig. 155A). If two workers are to use the room together the minimum area should be half as large again, that is about 6 feet by 12 or 7 feet by 10 (Fig. 155B). The layout should allow for a making-up bench down the longest side with plenty of shelves above and storage space below. A grinding bench should be across the short end furthest away from the door. A full-length window over the making-up bench and a smaller window on the opposite side or, better still over the grinding bench, is desirable to give cross-illumination. Any artificial lights should not throw the shadow of the worker onto the bench or the grinder. An extractor fan is almost a necessity to prevent a build-up of ammonia fumes from latex or of solvents from adhesives. A sink, with tap and waste, is desirable at the opposite end from the grinder so that impressions can be conveniently filled with plaster of paris. The room is best designed so that impressions come in on the plaster side by the sink, are filled there and placed on the plaster bench alongside. Casts are removed

from the impression compound when hard and any trimming necessary is done at that end of the room. When ready they are placed on
the long processing bench for making-up. When this is done they
are passed to the end nearest the grinder. After grinding they are
placed on shelves or racks to await trial fitting. Some people like to
have a hot air oven available to dry off wet casts and leathers. The
best place for this is on or under the processing bench in such a

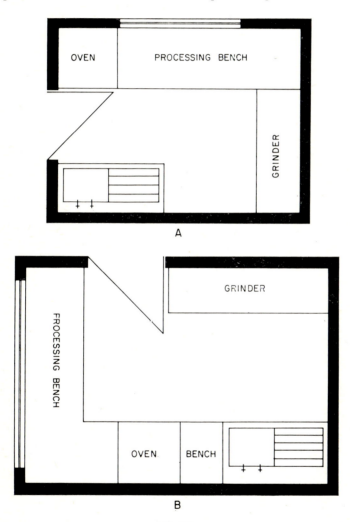

FIG. 155

Suggested plans for private practice appliance rooms: (A) six feet by
eight; (B) ten feet by seven.

position as to be accessible from the plaster bench as well as the making-up surface of the processing bench.

The choice of grinder is best left to the operator as he will know the purposes for which he wishes to use it, but some indication as to the types available and the purposes for which they are suitable will be found useful. The power and type of grinder needed naturally varies according to the nature of the bulk of the work to be done on it. Heavy work requires a powerful motor and although this will cope with lighter jobs its power makes it less suitable for them. Light grinders, on the other hand, cannot be expected to cope with heavy work or long runs.

The lightest type of grinder that can be used with any degree of success is the home workshop type of electric drill mounted on its bench stand and fitted with a drum sander. The $\frac{5}{16}$ inch drill size is needed and should have a power rating of at least 300 watts and speed of nearly 4000 revolutions per minute. It should not be subjected to long runs under load nor be heavily overloaded for short periods as the armature of this light type of motor soon over-heats and I have heard of one which has been burned out. For intermittent use, and if used with care, even for the occasional heavy job they perform amazingly well.

The next type is the double-ended bench grinder. The smallest of these has about the same power as the $\frac{5}{16}$ inch electric drill but, although it lacks the drill's versatility, the possession of double bearings and two grinding heads is a distinct advantage. Larger sizes of bench grinder can be obtained and those with a power rating of from one-third to one horsepower are very suitable indeed for our work. I have used one very satisfactorily for several years now. It is known as an 8 inch bench grinder and has a power rating in the neighbourhood of one horsepower. It is double-ended and fitted on one side with a 4 inch sole grinder (4 inches wide and 4 inches diameter) and, on the other side, with a $1\frac{1}{4}$ inch curved grinding wheel, ($1\frac{1}{4}$ inches wide and 6 inches in diameter with a slightly convex surface). These wheels are armoured with emery cloths (grit 60) of appropriate widths. This is a robust grinder and is rated for continuous use. It gets rather warm when used on long runs or on heavy work but has never given any trouble. There is no need for any speed variation as its steady 3950 revolutions per minute can cope satisfactorily with any work we are likely to use it for.

Some people will prefer to employ a one-third or one-half horse-power motor with a belt drive and short piece of shafting to take the grinders. It is usual to use multiple pulleys on the drive so that a variety of speeds may be obtained by presetting the driving belt onto any pair of pulleys. To allow of this the motor is usually mounted on a hinged flap the lifting of which slackens the belt and allows the driving ratios to be changed. When the flap is lowered the belt is tightened, and the weight of the motor keeps it tight ensuring good adhesion for the drive. Grinders can be mounted on the short shaft between external bearers and one end of the shaft can be threaded to take a chuck as an added refinement. The individual items comprising this type of grinder can often be picked up quite cheaply from time to time. Little skill is needed to assemble them and any good tool shop will advise as to the most suitable pulleys, shafting and bearings. The capacitor start motor is to be preferred and a proper starting switch must be used. If much grinding is to be done a dust hood is needed. This is erected around and behind the grinding wheels and is an attempt to catch most of the dust but it must be admitted that turbulence from the grinding wheels scatters the dust. The addition of suction is not as effective as one might hope. The hood has to be so large to encompass the grinders that air speed through it is greatly reduced and unless the suction is very powerful it will not overcome the turbulence. I have used some of the more powerful types of vacuum cleaners for this purpose but not, I fear, very satisfactorily.

Some people like to house their grinders in cabinets with a top which shuts down when not in use. When open the top forms part of the dust-trapping mechanism.

For the large workshop or professional appliance laboratory there is nothing to beat a simple adaptation of the shoe repairer's finishing machine. These machines have ample power both for the drive and the suction. The alteration is merely a reduction in the number of finishing wheels and the inclusion of a 4 inch sole grinder and a $1\frac{1}{4}$ inch curved and a $1\frac{1}{4}$ inch flat grinder. The Naumkeag head, if fitted, is best retained as it makes an excellent grinder for shaping small sponge rubber pads and the heated edge finisher finds use as an edge turner and finisher. The price of these machines precludes their use in most private practices but they are probably the best machines for this work.

17

Leathers used in Appliance Work

FOR those unfamiliar with the leathers used in appliance making the following brief notes are appended.

Leather is classified according to the animal from which it is obtained, the methods by which it is tanned and finished, and whether or not it is split or is of full thickness. The first point requires little elaboration except to say that nearly all chamois leathers originate from sheep or lambskins and not the chamois, and the term chamois leather is now taken to mean a method of tannage rather than an animal or origin.

The method of tannage is important as it affects the subsequent properties and finish of the leathers and to a certain extent governs their use. Tanning is a method whereby skins and hides are rendered imputrescent. The term skin applies more to small animals like sheep, lambs and goats whilst hide is used to denote larger skins such as those from horses, cattle (cows and oxen) and buffalo. Tanning not only makes the leather durable by preventing rotting, but improves its quality by rendering it more resistant to friction and scuffing, more flexible and easier to handle when making up into leather goods. It also makes leather more acceptable in use and better able to take dyes and finishes.

The traditional method of tannage consists of immersing a de-haired and defatted hide in a pit of water with vegetable products containing natural tannin, often for many months. The most important of these vegetable products is oak bark, but many other barks are employed as well as the twigs, leaves and fruits of many different trees and shrubs. The leathers so tanned are mostly of a fawn or brown colour in their natural state, i.e. unless dyed.

Chemical tannage has now become of great importance and consists of steeping the hides in a solution of chromium salts which tan the leather. This form of tannage is well adapted for use in hot countries where the hides putrefy quickly. This is a more rapid method than vegetable tannage and gives a more open type of leather which, since it takes wax polishes very well, is used extensively in the shoe trade for the making of uppers.

The only other form of tannage of any importance to us is that used for chamois leather. Here sheepskins are tanned by means of 'chamoising oils'. These are fish oils, mainly from the cod liver, and the process involves oxidation of the oil in the skin. It is this process which gives it its soft and slightly greasy feel as well as its yellow colour.

The outer surface of the hide, from which the hair and epidermis have been removed by a process of liming and scraping, is known as the grain side whereas the inner surface is termed the flesh side. Many hides are too thick for the use to which they are to be put so they are split into several layers. The layer bearing the grain surface is the grain split or skiver and that bearing the flesh surface is termed the flesh split. Suedes are leathers finished on the flesh side with a fine nap. With sheepskins the grain split is usually known as skiver and the flesh split as lining.

A leather very much used in chiropodial orthopædic work is sheepskin specially selected for surgical appliance work. The soft natural finish skin, known as natural surgical basil, is a wholly vegetable-tanned unsplit sheepskin left without dyeing. This is used mainly as the foundation leather of insoles made to a plaster cast. When wetted it stretches well over the cast and the grain surface provides a durable upper surface to the appliance. The various compounds used for making up the insole also bond to the flesh side well. The finished appliances are often covered, top and bottom, with surgical skiver. This, of course, is also a sheepskin.

Natural surgical Persians are semi-chrome-tanned leathers from Indian sheepskins tanned in India. They are soft and mould easily, so are used for covering replaceable plantar pads which are attached to the foot with elastic bands. They can also be used to replace chamois leather except where the pad comes in actual contact with the skin. They have a grain surface, which chamois lacks, and so wear better.

Chrome lambskins are unsplit lamb or sheepskin, chrome-tanned and with a soft grain. This is really a gloving leather which can be used as an alternative to the natural surgical Persian leather.

Natural calf is a vegetable-tanned leather made from the young ox or cow. It is usually stronger and thicker than natural surgical basil and, for our work, has little advantage over it.

Chamois leather is an oil-tanned, suede-finished leather made from the flesh split of sheep or lambskins. It is used for lining or covering pads which are placed on the skin or are worn inside the hosiery. Such pads may be washed carefully from time to time in warm water with soap but must be dried naturally and slowly. They must always be well powdered in wear.

All the leathers mentioned so far are relatively thin and flexible. There are times, however, when thicker and stronger leather is required. The first of these is flesher or fleshing leather. This is a coarse fibrous leather of loose texture from the inner or flesh side of a hide. In order to make it firmer, stronger and closer in texture it is filled by dipping in hot paraffin wax and rolling. This is a cheap leather used for the making of insole patterns of a shoe upon which can be mounted sponge or felt pads. As it is not of uniform thickness and it is difficult, owing to its high wax content, to adhere the pads and covering leathers to it, it is falling into disuse. Its place is being taken by sheets of synthetic material such as Regen and Cortex.

Strapping leather, sometimes called bridle shoulders, is a strong flexible leather of reasonably uniform thickness of 1–2 mm, with a plain finish and close-shaved flesh. It is made from ox or cow hide, vegetable-tanned and subject to a series of processes applied to the leather after tanning, in the course of which appropriate amounts of oils and greases are incorporated in the leather to give it increased tensile strength, flexibility and water-resisting qualities. It is used in our work for the soles of moccasin appliances as it is firm and flexible yet resists creasing and working back in the shoe. It is particularly useful where a toe-block prosthesis is incorporated in the moccasin. The oils and greases are, at times, a disadvantage and the flesh side has to be roughened and washed with methyl ether before good adhesion can be obtained to the chamois upper and sponge rubber infilling.

Blocking or moulding shoulder leather is that portion of the cattle hide covering the animals' shoulders. It is a light-weighing un-bleached bark-tanned leather. The thickness required is from 1.5 to 2.5 mm. This leather when soaked for about twenty-four hours in water is tacked onto the plaster cast of a foot and, by a process of beating with a light hammer or rolling and pressing with a smooth piece of wood such as a hammer handle or a lick stick, is moulded into the contours of the cast. When dry it will resist deformation to a very great extent but to ensure that the close fit is not lost in wear it is backed with a paste compounded of leather dust, granulated cork and wood flour bound with latex (p. 149). Blocking shoulder leather is particularly useful for making the double-flanged and cradle types of inlay as the firmness of the leather ensures that the flanges are not trodden down in wear.

DIRECTORY OF SUPPLIERS OF
APPLIANCE MATERIALS

B.D.H. (Woolley & Arnfield) Ltd Brinksway Road, P.O. Box 4 Stockport Cheshire	Plaster of paris Plaster of paris bandage (Gypsona) Spatulas
Charlesworth Shoe Company 6 John Dalton Street Manchester 2	Charlesworth Shoes
P. K. Dutt Ltd Clan Works Howard Lane Bromley Kent	Revertex, 60 per cent. centrifugal latex
Expanded Plastics Ltd Worple Road Isleworth Middlesex	Polythene Sheet Vitrithine
Expanded Rubber and Plastics Ltd Mitcham Road Croydon, Surrey	Rubberzote
Footman & Co Ltd 124/126 Haydons Road London S.W.19	Cortex Surgical Elastic Fine pink elastic net Lastonet Latex sheet
J. O. Grant & Co Ltd Timber Merchants Frederick Road Salford 6	Wood flour, 60's, 90's and 120's
Grundy's Rubber Ltd 11 Bridge Street West Manchester 3	Latex sheet (strip rubber): 15–20 thousandths of an inch thick Latex foam Latafoam Surgical sponge—sponge rubber Rubberzote closed cell

G. W. Hargreaves Ltd
43 Shudehill
Manchester 4
	All leathers Eyelets and
	                                              eyeletter
	All adhesives { Gripso Ring punch
	              Gripsotite Leather knives
	              Phillosol Emery cloths
	Pochin's Flexadhesive and solvent
	Pochin's bottom filler

Noel Hulme 268 Wellington Road South Stockport Cheshire	Dental superfine Plaster of paris
I.C.I. Silicone Rubbers Nobel Division Stevenston Ayrshire	Silicone rubbers

T

James Johnson Dale Street Works Milnrow Rochdale, Lancs.	Cork sheet Cork wedges (bevelled strip) Granulated cork
S. M. Ketteridge 52 Moorfield Road Salford 6	Hessian (scrim)
Midland Silicones Ltd Reading Bridge House Reading Berkshire	Silicone Rubber No. 2427 and Catalyst No. N.2428 (Cold Cure Silastomer)
Modern Loratex Products Inc. 88 Henry Street Binghamton New York, U.S.A.	Molo
Mushpro Ltd 2a Ashdown Street London N.W.5	Disposable plastic gloves
Wm. R. Pangbourne & Sons Leather Manufacturers & Merchants Bounds Green London N.11	All leathers including: Basils Splits Skivers Strapping Chamois Oak bark blocking shoulder and belly leathers
Portland Plastics Hythe Kent	Disposable plastic gloves
Rubber Latex Ltd Harling Road Wythenshawe Manchester 22	Pre-vulcanised latex
Surgical Supply Service 825 Walnut Street Philadelphia Pa. U.S.A.	Molo
The S. S. White Dental Mfg. Co (G.B.) Ltd 126 Great Portland Street London W.1 and provincial depots	Dental wax Alginate casting compound Rubber plaster bowls

Index

Index